Enhancing Human Performance in Sport: New Concepts and Developments

American Academy
of Physical Education Papers
No. 25

ENHANCING HUMAN PERFORMANCE IN SPORT: NEW CONCEPTS AND DEVELOPMENTS

American Academy of Physical Education Papers No. 25

Sixty-Third Annual Meeting
San Francisco, California
April 2-3, 1991

Published by Human Kinetics Publishers
for the American Academy of Physical Education

Editors
Robert W. Christina
Helen M. Eckert

Academy Seal designed by
R. Tait McKenzie

Managing Editor: Julia Anderson
Copyeditor: Peg Goyette
Typesetter: Julie Overholt

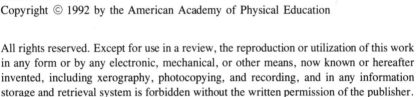

ISBN 0-87322-353-5
ISSN 0741-4633
Copyright © 1992 by the American Academy of Physical Education

Library of Congress Cataloging-in-Publication Data

Enhancing human performance in sport : new concepts and developments.
    p.   cm. -- (American Academy of Physical Education papers,
ISSN 0741-4633 ; no. 25)
   Papers from the Sixty-third Annual Meeting of the American Academy of Physical Education.
   Includes bibliographical references.
   ISBN 0-87322-353-5
   1. Sports sciences--Congresses. 2. Performance--Congresses.
I. American Academy of Physical Education.   II. Series.
GV557.5.E54 1992   91-47623
613.7'1--dc20   CIP

Printed in the United States of America
3 2 1

Human Kinetics Books
A Division of Human Kinetics Publishers,
  Inc.
Box 5076, Champaign, IL 61825-5076
1-800-747-4457

Canada Office:
Human Kinetics Publishers, Inc.
P.O. Box 2503, Windsor, ON N8Y 4S2
1-800-465-7301 (in Canada only)

Europe Office:
Human Kinetics Publishers (Europe) Ltd.
P.O. Box IW14
Leeds LS19 6TR
England
(0532) 781708

CONTENTS

Enhancing Human Performance in Sport: An Introduction

Robert W. Christina
State University of New York at Buffalo

The theme of this volume of *The Academy Papers* is "Enhancing Human Performance in Sport: New Concepts and Developments." With the immense popularity of sport and exercise in recent years, and with all that is being publicized, the theme of the Sixty-third Annual Meeting of the American Academy of Physical Education and this volume seemed very timely and appropriate. The program emanating from this theme was developed in order to identify, discuss, and evaluate some of the new concepts and developments for enhancing human performance in sport. It also was designed with the intention of going beyond these boundaries in order to examine and reflect on the broad implications of applying these concepts and developments to enhance human performance in sport.

Eight major papers focusing on the theme and eight reactions to these papers are included in this volume. Authors of the major papers were asked to prepare their manuscripts from their own academic perspective and area of expertise. The areas they represent include history, biomechanics, motor learning, motor development, sport sociology, sport psychology, exercise physiology, and philosophy. When preparing their manuscripts, authors were asked to consider the following questions:

1. What are new concepts and developments in your area?
2. How do these new concepts and developments enhance performance in sport?
3. What scientific evidence is there to indicate that the new concepts and developments actually enhance performance in sport?
4. Who will be able to use these new concepts and developments, and in what context (if not obvious)?
5. What are the tradeoffs or cost-benefit factors of using the new concepts and developments?
6. What are the broad implications of using the new concepts and developments?

It is hoped that the following articles will acquaint readers with some of the new concepts and developments that have emerged from the various exercise and sport sciences. It is also hoped that these papers will stimulate thinking about and the evaluation the "cutting edge" ideas, practices, techniques, and issues that in recent years have been central to the enhancement of human performance in sport.

A Historical Look at Enhancement of Performance in Sport: Muscular Moralists Versus Muscular Scientists

Ronald A. Smith
Penn State University

If it took me over a decade to research and write a history of the first half-century of big-time intercollegiate athletics in America, it would be presumptuous to try to present a history of the enhancement of performance in sport in a few months. It seemed an impossible task when Bob Christina asked me to do it, but I agreed. I did so because I owed Bob a favor. A couple years ago after an AAHPERD convention, Bob asked me to play golf in Las Vegas at one of the pro tour stops. Just being in the same foursome with Bob was an honor. I now return the golfing favor which, incidentally, cost me $85 just to get on the course, not including what I lost during the match. Thanks, Bob.

Historically, many leading physical educators have been opposed to the enhancement of human performance at the upper levels of athletic participation. Historically, physical educators in America have been *least* interested in studying the Bob Christinas, who have extreme skill in sports such as golf, and more interested in those who lack the basic skills—the Rodney Dangerfields of physical abilities.

This has interested me, since I came into the profession through the back door. After earning two degrees in history, I entered a doctoral program in physical education at the University of Wisconsin. The first paper I did in physical education was a bit of independent historical research into an aspect of the medical and scientific background of Dudley Sargent, Luther Gulick, Clark Hetherington, and R. Tait McKenzie. I was interested to find that there was a strong antipathy toward star athletes—to those, they said, who needed physical activity the least.

Later I came across two individuals born in the 19th century who had just the opposite view, Pierre de Coubertin and George Santayana. Coubertin probably does not need much of an introduction to you, except to dismiss the myth that he created the modern Olympics. He didn't, but he did internationalize the Games, which the Greeks themselves had resurrected beginning in 1859.[1] Coubertin did introduce other nations into the 1896 Games in Athens. However, he made a point about the need to emphasize excellence in athletic performance and to accent those who were the best. Coubertin stated,

> In order for a hundred people to take part in physical culture, it is necessary for fifty to take part in sport; in order for fifty to take part in sport, twenty must specialize; in order for twenty to specialize, five must be capable of astonishing feats of prowess.[2]

Coubertin believed that if we desire mass participation in exercise and sport, we need a showcase of the talented.

George Santayana, the great Harvard philosopher of the late 1800s, made a slightly different point in an interesting article published in 1894. In an eclectic essay, titled "Philosophy on the Bleachers," Santayana called for an "athletic aristocracy," one that would reach heights in sport that few could ever realize. Santayana said there is an athletic aristocracy for the same reason that there is one of intelligence: because individuals have different endowments and only a few can do something as well as the activity is capable of being done. Then Santayana wrote,

> The value of talent, the beauty and dignity of positive achievements, depend on the height reached, and not on the number that reach it. Only the supreme is interesting: the rest has value only as leading to it or reflecting it.[3]

So, like Coubertin, Santayana saw excellence in sport as leading others to its enjoyment, both as participants and as spectators.

If Coubertin and Santayana were correct, that mass participation in exercise and sport will be furthered by those who reach the peak in sport performance, it seems only logical that physical education professionals should want to scientifically study ways to reach sport excellence. Coubertin and Santayana did not directly say so, but they might have called our field the study of exercise and sport science—a most logical name.

Why did our profession take another direction away from the study of high performance? Why did early 20th-century male leaders, such individuals as Dudley Allen Sargent, Clark Hetherington, and Luther Gulick, and especially female leaders such as Senda Berenson, Mabel Lee, Delphine Hanna, and Lucille Eaton Hill, oppose the study of high level athletes? Wellesley's Lucille Hill may have stated it best when in 1903 she said that sports should contribute the "greatest good to the greatest number, not the greatest good to the smallest number."[4]

Taking the cue from leaders such as Hill, it is not likely that others in women's physical education would be interested in studying the highest levels of women's sports. If women opposed higher levels of competition such as intercollegiate competition at any skill level, they would hardly want to study the elite performers.

Male physical educators often took a similar stance. Dudley Allen Sargent was not well liked at Harvard over the years, in part because he was strongly opposed to elite athletes. His participation on the faculty athletic committee at Harvard beginning in 1882 was abhorred by both the general student body and the athletes because they believed he put obstacles in the way of producing winners. Sargent, highly trained as a professional circus performer and later as a medical doctor, often spoke out against highly talented athletes.

In 1906, when he was fighting for his professional life at Harvard and President Eliot was asking why no Harvard athletes saw any value in physical education, Sargent revealed his true feelings about Harvard athletes. After 25 years at Harvard, Sargent said that "at least one of Harvard's former athletes has come to appreciate the educational value of physical culture." That is about right, for most other athletes at Harvard detested Sargent for not being supportive of intercollegiate athletics. Because of Sargent's beliefs, you can understand why. He continued, in his reply to President Eliot, that for athletes at Harvard there is the

> pursuit of athletics as an end rather than a means to an end, i.e. the giving of spectacles, shows and expensive amusements by a small number of experts to please the crowd, rather than to improve the mental and physical condition of the largest number of participants.[5]

Is it any wonder that those who followed in the steps of Lucille Eaton Hill at Wellesley and Dudley Allen Sargent at Harvard often took up the cudgel in opposition to the study of the highly skilled athlete or the enhancement of performance in sport? It was bred into our profession from the top down—a trickle-down principle. It has taken us a century to rectify the situation. Though there are still those who follow the precepts of the Hills and the Sargents, we are finally free of guilt when we study the best in order to enhance the performance, or to understand it, not only of the elite but of all those who might benefit from exercise and sport.

The profession had many medical doctors as leaders but few were interested in science. There were too few George Fitzes, who were both interested in and capable of doing research. Even Fitz, a professor of physiology and hygiene at Harvard, was nearly fired at one point in his career for lack of publications. As some of you know, Fitz in 1891 began the first bachelor's degree program in physical education at Harvard. His physiological laboratory was part of the Harvard Scientific School, and it never attracted many students; only nine graduated in the years between 1891 and 1899. Fitz wrote in 1893,

> Little has been done in the physiological and psychological effects of exercise. . . . Those engaged in the work have been too involved in the practical side, or too little versed in the exact physiological methods, to give much time to the less tangible aspects of exercise.[6]

Fitz's curiosity led him to raise questions about athletic performance: "Why is one boy a better catcher behind the bat, or able to hit the ball surer in tennis and baseball?" "What will give the best muscular development?" He wanted to answer some of the questions in his physiological laboratory. Unfortunately, even Fitz nearly lost his job because of the lack of publishing.

Ellen Gerber, in her book titled *Innovators and Institutions in Physical Education*, claimed that Fitz was "a prolific writer and speaker . . . [whose research was] published in professional, medical and scientific journals," yet he was nearly released by President Eliot.[7] After 8 years as assistant professor, he responded to Eliot's charge that he had failed "to publish the results of original work." Fitz tried to justify his lack of publishing and stated in a letter to President Eliot, "Day after day and week after week, I have not had an hour for original work free from imperative interruptions."[8]

Harvard's Eliot would not let up on Fitz or on Dudley Allen Sargent. After listening to a speech by Sargent at which Eliot said that his "mind rather slaggered as [Sargent] read," Eliot commented that recreation should not be a duty, it should be enjoyable. Eliot took the floor, criticizing Sargent and at the same time challenging George Fitz and Dr. Bowditch of the medical faculty to determine whether reaction time could be improved with practice. "Now, that is a rather elementary state of ignorance it seems to me," Eliot claimed, "after all the attention which has been given to psychology and to the training of the body."[9]

At the time possibly more research was being conducted by practitioners, coaches, and trainers in the field than by the leading physical educators. Why? Because coaches wanted to know how performance could be maximized whereas most physical educators were not interested in the performance of elite athletes. As an example, I have chosen two very successful coaches from a win/loss standpoint. The first, Charles Courtney, was a longtime coach of the Cornell crew from the 1880s to the 1910s. Courtney was a fine amateur photographer who, according to an observer of the time, used "his camera a great deal in pointing out to the men just what their faults are."[10] So one might say that Courtney was doing his own biomechanical analysis through photography.

Another coach, Bill Reid of Harvard, was doing film analysis of football kicking in 1905, the same year that Dudley Allen Sargent was railing against the pursuit of athletics as an end in itself. Reid used photos of himself and Percy Haughton, another great punter, to show to those on the Harvard team who were attempting to improve their skill in the kicking game.[11]

The same year that Reid was attempting to improve football skill through film analysis, the team physician was conducting his own research on athletic injuries of Harvard football players. Here again is something that Sargent, a medical doctor, might have done as head of physical education at Harvard. But Sargent was more interested in banning football than in studying it in any scientific manner. Edward Nichols, the Harvard team physician, carefully studied injuries during the 1905 season. Afterward, the results were published in the *Boston Medical and Surgical Journal*.[12]

The article contributed to the increased denouncing of intercollegiate football and called for a reform of the rules to help reduce the number of football injuries. Three months after the article was published, the football rules committee did indeed open the game up by allowing the forward pass for the first time. Dr. Nichols' research might have had something to do with the needed reform.

The fact that Sargent, the physical educator, sat idly by while others were doing research on high-performance athletes was symbolic of the profession, for most physical educators with medical degrees—the leaders of the profession— were doing the same. Harvard's George Fitz, who has never been adequately recognized by the physical education profession, was doing some research work with top-level athletes. He was studying varsity crew members, particularly their food consumption, calories, and excretion to determine the nitrogen intake and outgo. In 1898, he stated that it was "very possible that the men eat far more of the nitrogenous food than is needed, and that it may act harmfully is at least a possibility."[13]

Fitz might have contributed a great deal more scientifically had he not been involved in teaching courses in hygiene, physiology, and anatomy as well as being in charge of student health and having over 2,000 medical visits with students each year.[14] Besides this, he became founding editor of the *American*

Physical Education Review, the predecessor to *Research Quarterly* and the *Journal of Physical Education, Recreation and Dance*. In addition, Fitz became corresponding secretary of the American Association for the Advancement of Physical Education and was elected president of the Physical Education Section of the National Education Association.[15]

One might speculate that Harvard, the first institution to grant a bachelors degree in physical education, might have continued to do so had Dudley Allen Sargent given it more support and produced more scientific work. (To his credit, Sargent did teach an anthropometry course in the program.) Yet he may have felt that the physical education program in the Harvard Scientific School was in direct competition with his own private Sargent School for Physical Education and his famed Harvard Summer School of Physical Education.[16]

A few other medically trained physical educators did some research on highly skilled athletes. One was George L. Meylan of Columbia University, who did a study on longevity of former Harvard rowers. In addition to longevity, he also wanted to know whether crew members tended to be sterile, because of vigorous athletics, than men who were not intensively involved in competitive sports. Meylan found that not only did crew members live longer but that they were *not* more sterile than nonrowers.[17]

Both Meylan and Fitz were members of the American Society for Research in Physical Education, but Fitz soon became disillusioned with research efforts on high-performance athletics. For a decade and a half his charge to the profession essentially went unheard. "What we need is scientific work," he wrote in 1892, "not the assumption that certain laws require certain exercises. . . . I, too, see the dawn of the day. . . . It will come when we have the equal study of physiology and physical training."[18] By 1906 Fitz, opposed to the nonscientific trends in physical education, dropped out of the profession and went into private medical practice. The profession lost one of its finest early scientific investigators. Study of performance would have to come primarily from outside the field of physical education for the next half century.

The medical doctors who moved physical education from the late 19th century into the 20th century were principally "muscular moralists," not "muscular scientists." Men and women in the profession were more concerned with what they considered moral rightness than with physical performance, especially high-level performance. For instance, members of the Athletic Research Society, founded in the early 1900s by physical educators and others interested in athletics, were much more concerned with what they considered moral issues, such as preserving amateurism, than with athletes' diets or knowledge of the circulatory system in exercise.

Even a person as great as R. Tait McKenzie was more interested in the ancient Greek term *aidos* than in *aretê*. *Aidos* is the quality of honorableness and fairness in competition. *Aretê* is the desire for excellence in all things. These are two fine qualities, but physical educators such as R. Tait McKenzie were much more interested in the one than the other.[19] Now I am not opposed to those who favor *aidos* over *aretê*, but it has had a rather large negative effect upon our fundamental knowledge of performance and led to a lack of scientific research in our field historically. This, I suggest, contributed to the low status of physical educators among scholars in general.

The fact that Dudley Sargent at Harvard and Delphine Hanna at Oberlin College collected a lot of anthropometric data does not mean that they had true scientific minds. Their data generally sat in collective silence, as did most other anthropometric data in our field, though it made us look and feel somewhat scientific. However, Sargent's anthropometric research results at Harvard did provide R. Tait McKenzie with the data to sculpt his famous "The Ideal College Athlete."[20] Not everything was lost through anthropometry. Nevertheless, the collection of anthropometric measures did little to answer fundamental questions of performance.

One could argue that the Athletic Research Society of the early 1900s delayed scientific research because those in it generally favored the value-laden goals of sport and were little involved in value-free research. Those who favored the true amateur spirit in sport would almost never emphasize the scientific study of sport, for this would rationalize and professionalize the process of producing winners. This muscular moralist attitude in the physical education profession delayed scientific research. It led to a lack of disciplinary research and had a negative impact on our profession that is still felt.

By the 1920s and 1930s, physical education was led by the likes of Mabel Lee and Jesse Feiring Williams, neither of whom were scientifically oriented. Both Lee and Williams were researchers in a superficial sense. Both knew the answers to their research before they did it. Mabel Lee's famed but biased article, written in 1923, has been one of the most important in women's sport history. Titled "The Case For and Against Intercollegiate Athletics for Women and the Situation as it Stands Today," her article contained data of questionable validity to prove the point she wanted to make. Lee's point was to show emphatically how much women were opposed to competitive sports for women.[21]

That attitude was promulgated without any adequate research to prove that high-level athletic competition for women was harmful to them. The attitude of opposing interscholastic, intercollegiate, and Olympic level competition was foisted upon the entire profession of women physical educators by those in leadership positions for the next generation.[22] Lee was still opposing it in 1983 when, in her 90s, she wrote *A History of Physical Education and Sports in the U.S.A.* Still railing against highly competitive athletics, she recorded in her introduction, "I have tried to keep 'quack' amateur sports [i.e., intercollegiate athletics] in their correct place."[23]

The tendency for women to eschew scientific research in the performance domain has been evidenced in the literature. In the 1980s Christine Wells had to admit that there was still little collected knowledge about women athletes. As she said at an Academy meeting, "There is really very little strength data available from women athletes. . . . We really don't know the lower limit for [women's] body fat. . . . The same problems are encountered when we consider anaerobic power."[24]

It was the same in men's physical education when the dominant forces were men like Jesse Feiring Williams. Williams, who said that "Cultivation of the body for the body's sake can never be justified," tended to override the thoughts of others that a study of athletic performance for its own sake was a worthy objective.[25] His ideas even overshadowed the more scientific research of Charles H. McCloy who, as much as any other physical educator of his time, exemplified understanding performance by being a muscular scientist rather than a muscular moralist like Williams.

Some of the more recent leaders in research in the discipline have felt the need to refrain from research of high-level athletic performance or hide the fact that they were once high-level performers themselves. It seems that our physical education professionals or exercise scientists have too often been embarrassed that we might have been intercollegiate athletes, or Olympians, or professional athletes.

I think it was unfortunate that my doctoral advisor at the University of Wisconsin, Gerald Kenyon, hid the fact that he had been a champion pole vaulter in Canada. That he had been a champion athlete should not have tarnished his image as a quality sport sociologist. It should have added to his stature, for among other reasons he was better able to understand sport from a competitive standpoint. We also should not be embarrassed about studying the best athletes in a variety of sport contexts. A 1922 Nobel laureate, A.V. Hill, may have said something important when he wrote in his book, *Muscular Movement in Man*, that studying athletes "may help to bring new and enthusiastic recruits," those athletes who have been studied, into the field of research.[26]

In the long run we could honor those in our profession who have done research in performance when it was not socially acceptable to do so. We should thank the George Fitzes and the Charles McCloys for leading against the tide who considered muscular morality to be the only domain of physical education. It may be that, but it is much more. Our history of enhancing performance through scientific study has not been an exemplary one.

One is reminded of an occurrence in the 1950s which might demonstrate that as physical educators we did not take the lead in areas we should have known best. Only 8 years after World War II, a medical doctor, Hans Kraus, was studying chronic back pain and decided to test American and European children to see whether they had enough abdominal strength to prevent chronic back pain as they got older. He found that less than 10% of European children between the ages of 6 and 13 failed a simple test of minimum strength and flexibility. By contrast, well over 50% of American children failed the minimum fitness test.[27] Where was the physical education profession?

Physical educators, after eight decades of professional organization and an emphasis on physical education in the schools, still did not know what the minimal levels of physical fitness were for our children. It took an outsider who was testing chronic back pain, and the president of the United States, Dwight Eisenhower, who created the President's Council on Physical Fitness and Youth,[28] to awaken us to the fact that scientific research into physical fitness was worthy of our collective attention. Then, when we did create a test of physical fitness, it was of questionable validity.

From a muscular scientific standpoint we had failed, and we were not quite sure from a muscular morality conviction whether we should give fitness the emphasis that the nation knew it needed. It was a shameful period in our profession's history.

The profession seemed out of tune with national needs and desires. And we were out of tune, from an international standpoint, with the need to be doing scientific studies in high-performance athletics. Whether physical educators wanted to study our elite athletes or not, it was in our national interest to do so. The

Cold War era, which created an immediate need for physically fit youth, also created the need for outstanding athletes who could perform at a level of excellence in international competitions such as the Olympics. Just as the international need to be physically fit was not being met by muscular moralists, who led the physical education profession, neither was the physical education profession conducting scientific studies to improve the performance of our best athletes to succeed at the international level.

The 1950s and 1960s saw the rise of disciplinary splinter groups, which began to break away from the American Association for Health, Physical Education and Recreation and the National College Physical Education Association for Men. The splintering was begun by exercise physiologists, but others soon followed. The splintering was done not by muscular moralists but by muscular scientists. Not until the splintering began was there a concerted effort by those in physical education to better understand performance. It was necessary to splinter into groups for the scientific and humanistic study of such areas as biomechanics, history, motor performance, philosophy, physiology, psychology, and sociology of sport.

It was probably important historically to have muscular moralists, those committed to the value of promoting physical activity for our youth. Thus the Senda Berensons and the Clark Hetheringtons served a useful purpose. But the muscular moralists failed to give real scholarly authenticity to our profession, for they were not actively involved in research that would be accepted by other scholars. Physical education lagged far behind other scholarly endeavors. It is not surprising that most of the work in exercise physiology was being done outside our field; that biomechanical discoveries were often generated by those not in physical education; that motor performance research was being conducted by those other than physical educators; that sport history was first done by historians, not physical educators.

Not enough muscular moralists saw the need for muscular scientists, and thus the leaders, the muscular moralists, hired other muscular moralists to continue their work. Not until they saw the need for the scholarly productivity and prestige that comes from muscular scientists were the scientists brought into the field in significant numbers. This began in earnest in the 1960s and has continued.

We can see the changes in the last generation in the makeup of the American Academy of Physical Education. Where once nearly every member was what I have defined as a muscular moralist, the trend in the last decade or two is toward the muscular scientist. That process has generated a great deal of discussion, including a possible name change of the American Academy of Physical Education. Today, those who want to advance the profession through the advancement of knowledge, what I have here called the muscular scientists, are in the ascendancy, and many of them are involved in research that will enhance all levels of physical performance. It has been a long historical process, but today we have some *aretê* with our *aidos*.

Notes

¹Young, D.C. (1987). The origins of the modern Olympics: A new version. *International Journal of the History of Sport*, **4**, 271-300.

[2]de Coubertin, P. (1966). The philosophic foundation of modern Olympism. *The Olympic idea* (pp. 131-132), Schorndorf, Germany: Druckerei und Verlag Karl Hofmann; de Coubertin, P. (1931). *Mémoires Olympiques* (pp. 217-218). Lausanne, Switzerland: Bureau International de Pedegogie Sportive.

[3]Santayana, G. (1894). Philosophy on the bleachers. *Harvard Monthly*, **8**, 181-190.

[4]Hill, L.E. (1903). *Athletic and outdoor sports for women*. New York: Macmillan.

[5]Sargent, D.A. (1906, April 26). Letter to Jerome D. Green, Secretary to President Charles Eliot, Harvard. Eliot Papers, Box 245, Folder "Sargent," Harvard University Archives.

[6]As quoted in Gerber, E.W. (1971). *Innovators and institutions in physical education* (p. 305). Philadelphia: Lea & Febiger.

[7]Ibid., pp. 395-396.

[8]Fitz, G.W. (1899, April 4). Letter to President Charles W. Eliot, Harvard. Eliot Papers, Box 136, Folder 1170, Harvard University Archives.

[9]Talk by Charles W. Eliot. (undated manuscript, c. 1900). Eliot Papers, Box 110, Folder 144, Harvard University Archives.

[10]*The Cornell Daily Sun*. (1893, June 26). p. 4.

[11]Reid, W.T., Jr. (1905). *1905 Football Diary* (vol. I). Harvard University Archives.

[12]Nichols, E.H., & Smith C. (1906, January 4). The physical aspect of American football. *Boston Medical and Surgical Journal*, **154**, 1-8.

[13]Fitz, G.W. (1898, November 28). Letter to President Charles W. Eliot, Harvard. Eliot Papers, Box 136, Folder 1170, Harvard University Archives.

[14]Fitz, G.W. (1899, April 4). Letter to President Charles W. Eliot, Harvard. Eliot Papers, Box 268, Folder "Mar–May 1899," Harvard University Archives.

[15]Fitz, G.W. (1899, May 28). Letter to President Charles W. Eliot, Harvard. Eliot Papers, Box 136, Folder 1170, Harvard University Archives.

[16]Gerber, E. (1971). In *Innovators and institutions in physical education* (pp. 304, 305). She notes that only once did Sargent ever mention the Harvard degree program in any of his writings.

[17]Meylan, G.L. (1904, March). Harvard University oarsmen. *Harvard Graduates' Magazine*, 362-376. This research was in concert with Dr. E.H. Bradford's 1878 findings that Harvard crew members lived longer than the general population. (See *Harvard Advocate*, January, 18, p. 100.) An earlier study in England of Oxford and Cambridge rowers showed that rowers' longevity was greater than nonathletic men. (See Blaikie, W. [1873]. Ten years among the rowing men. *Harper's Monthly*, **47**, 413.)

Park, R.J. (1990). *Athletes and their training in Britain and America, 1800-1914*. This unpublished manuscript notes that the English study was done by John Morgan, a physician who had been a former athlete, not by a physical educator.

For a review of athletic longevity, see Stephens, K.E., et al. (1983). The longevity, morbidity, and physical fitness of former athletes—an update. In H.M. Eckert & H.J. Montoye (Eds.), *American Academy of Physical Education Papers: Exercise and Health* (vol. 17), (pp. 101-120).

For more of the work of George L. Meylan, see Meylan, G.L. (1913). Athletic training. *American Physical Education Review*, **18**, 217-229.

[18]Gerber, E. (1971). *Innovators and institutions in physical education*, p. 302.

[19]McKenzie, R.T. (1911). The chronicle of the amateur spirit. *American Physical Education Review*, **16**, 79-94.

[20]McKenzie, R.T. (1910). *Exercise in education and medicine* (pp. 192-193). Philadelphia: Saunders.

[21]Lee, M. (1931). The case for and against intercollegiate athletics for women as it stands today. *Mind and Body*, **30**, 246-255. Her article a decade later (May 1931), "The case for and against intercollegiate athletics for women and the situation since 1923" (*Research Quarterly*, **2**, 16-31), is equally as biased.

[22]Gerber, E. The controlled development of collegiate sport for women, 1923–1936. *Journal of Sport History*, **2**, 1-28; Hult, J.S. (1985, Centennial Issue), The governance of athletics for girls and women: Leadership by women physical educators, 1889–1949. *Research Quarterly for Exercise and Sport*, 64-77; Lucas, J.A., & Smith, R.A. (1978). *Saga of American Sport* (pp. 342-372). Philadelphia: Lea & Febiger.

[23]Lee, M. (1983). *A history of physical education and sports in the U.S.A.* (p. vi). New York: Wiley & Sons.

[24]Wells, C.L. (1984). The limits of female performance. In D.A. Clarke & H.M. Eckert (Eds.), *American Academy of Physical Education Papers: Limits of Human Performance*, **18**, 84, 82, 85.

[25]Williams, J.F. (1932). *The principles of physical education* (p. 286). Philadelphia: Saunders.

[26]Montoye, H.J. (1984). The scientific study of athletes and athletics. *American Academy of Physical Education*, **18**, 2-3.

[27]Kraus, H, & Hirschland, R.P. (1953). Muscular fitness and health. *Journal of Health, Physical Education and Recreation*, **24**, 17-19.

[28]When Eisenhower initiated his conference on fitness and youth, 32 individuals were invited to the White House. None was a physical educator. None has ever chaired the President's Council on Physical Fitness and Sport. See Clarke, H. (1970). The president's address: Academy directions. In Donna May Miller & Elwood Frank Davis (Eds.), *American Academy of Physical Education Papers*, **4**, 69.

Why Moralists More Than Scientists? Reflections on Origins and Consequences

Roberta J. Park
University of California, Berkeley

Since I am in essential agreement with Professor Smith's paper, this reaction will focus upon two things: (a) a glimpse at some of the late 19th/early 20th century work of "muscular scientists," especially those associated with the field of physical education, and (b) an attempt to explain why the field, in general, took the "muscular moralist" path. At the close of my remarks, I will attempt to show that although developments since the 1960s have been on the whole salubrious, we are now fatally close to permitting scientism to unduly narrow our focus and restrict the potential that our field offers for advancing human understanding.

It is largely, but not wholly, accurate to say that early physical educators were disinterested in studying, much less enhancing, upper levels of human performance. Dr. Watson Savage (President of the American Physical Education Association from 1901 to 1903) and colleagues undertook extensive studies of the "Physiological and Pathological Effects of Severe Exertion" during the 1909 Pittsburgh Marathon Race.

They gathered biographical and medical data as well as anecdotal information about previous athletic experiences. They also collected data on weight loss, rectal temperature, heart size by means of X ray, condition of the heart immediately after and a week after the race, blood pressure, urinary samples, and other physiological measures. Indeed, the 1909 Pittsburgh Marathon was organized partly to collect such data (Barach, 1911; Savage, 1910).

There were two major motivations: (a) American Johnnie Hayes' victory in the marathon race at the 1908 London Olympic Games, and the ensuing interest in distance running, and (b) the more general interest in achieving a scientific understanding of circulation, metabolism, and other parameters of human performance which, although small, had been growing since the 1870s. Reports of Savage's findings were presented at the 1909 annual meetings of the College Gymnasium Director's Society and published as a six-part series in the *American Physical Education Review*.

Earlier Dr. Austin Flint Jr. (1878) had collected metabolic information during a 5-day 400-mile walk by the famous American pedestrian Edward Payson Weston. It was also in the 1870s that interest arose in studying the phenomenon of "the athlete's heart" (cf. Whorton, 1982). Among those researching such topics was Alfred Stengel, professor of clinical medicine at the University of Pennsylvania, who in 1899 published "The Immediate and Remote Effects of Athletics Upon the Heart and Circulation."

The impetus for improvements in athletic *performance*, however, came substantially from trainers and coaches such as Michael Murphy (1894; 1914), who served at Yale and then at the University of Pennsylvania. Murphy, who became one of America's preeminent track coaches, had studied medicine for 2 years. For the most part, however, men who served as trainers relied more on experience and observing outstanding athletes than on clinical or experimental research.

Among the early APEA members who expressed considerable interest in exploring the limits of human performance was George Wells Fitz, a man now largely forgotten in the history of the profession. While serving as director of the nation's first 4-year academic degree program in anatomy, physiology, and physical training at Harvard University between 1892 and 1898, Fitz (1893, 1895) conducted investigations of reaction time, asking, for example, "How do humans accurately control their muscles in their infinitely complicated combination?" Such questions were of practical as well as scientific interest, he observed, as they related to issues like why one boy was a "better catcher behind the bat, or able to hit the ball surer in tennis and baseball" (Fitz, 1893, p. 27).

There is archival evidence that Fitz also had intended to conduct circulatory and metabolic studies on the Harvard crew team, but the termination of his position at Harvard after the 1898 academic year resulted in these being carried out by Eugene Darling, MD (1899, 1901). In passing, we might note that Darling took the bulk of Fitz's 4-year program in anatomy, physiology, and physical training as the basis for the new program in anatomy, physiology, and hygiene that was offered by Harvard's Lawrence Scientific School in 1901—expunging everything that had to do with "physical training."

James H. McCurdy (1901) investigated the effect of maximal muscular effort on blood pressure, reporting his findings in the *American Journal of Physiology*. Wilbur Bowen (1903a,b) conducted various studies of the effects of muscular work on the pulse rate. APEA member Dr. James A. Babbitt (1901) examined the influence of athletics and gymnastic exercise on hemoglobin. Naval surgeon Henry G. Beyer, an early member of the AAAPE and a founding member of the American Physiological Society, analyzed the height, weight, lung capacity, and strength of Annapolis cadets between 1892 and 1894. Using his own data and similar information collected at Yale and Amherst, Beyer (1894) concluded that systematic gymnastic drills and rowing were more conducive to all-around development than was football.

In the early 1900s, the American Association for Advancement of Science included four papers pertaining to exercise and physical training as part of Section K, "Physiology and Experimental Medicine." In addition to addresses by physicians R. Tait McKenzie and Thomas Storey, APEA member Theodore Hough (1909), then professor of physiology at the University of Virginia, and Frederic S. Lee (1909), professor of physiology at Columbia University, presented papers dealing with physical exercise, katabolism, and fatigue.

Introducing his paper, Hough (1909) made a clear, and on the whole unbiased, distinction between physical training and athletics. For the former, the object was "to secure for each individual student the proper basis of health for his work in school or college and also to educate him in the truest sense of that word for the proper hygienic conduct of his subsequent life." The athletic ideal, on the other hand, was not primarily concerned with "cultivation of health but [with] excelling someone else" (p. 484). Indeed, the athlete must be ready to incur risks to prove himself superior.

Hough did not reject the athletic ideal, nor did he believe it was necessarily inferior to the hygienic orientation. He did ask, however, that one be clear that although both involved the same physiological processes, their purposes were markedly different. His particular interest, not surprisingly, was with "the biological requirements of the human body for muscular activity as an essential factor in health (p. 485).

It is not necessary to look far afield to grasp why Hough and the vast majority of turn-of-the-century physical educators adhered, in varying ways, to the hygienic as opposed to the athletic ideal. The motivations were several, but the three most significant can aptly be described as the altruistic/reform impulse, biomedical considerations, and the search for professional legitimacy.

Many turn-of-the-century Americans adhered to strong and lingering currents of the antebellum "health reform" movement (cf. Green, 1986; Whorton, 1982). At its more extreme, this had seen wholesome, robust health as something tantamount to the millennium. By the 1870s, millennial zeal was rapidly giving way to the "social reform" impulses that swept the nation from the centennial celebrations of 1876 through the Progressive Era.

Given these interests and persuasions, it should not be surprising that health, exercise, and physical training formed part of several annual programs of the American Social Science Association in the 1870s and 1880s, before the AAAPE was founded. Both Edward M. Hartwell (1880) and Dudley Allen Sargent (1884), early AAAPE presidents and leaders of the emerging field, gave papers at ASSA meetings in the 1880s. So did Dr. Grace Peckham (1887), the neurologist Dr. James Putnam (1876), and Dr. D.F. Lincoln (1876), a member of the AAAPE in the 1890s.

Both Putnam and Lincoln were respected New England physicians; both had spent time abroad studying medicine at one of the German universities. Indeed, the late and wide-ranging 19th-century biomedical interest in exercise and physical training was clearly associated with reasons why so many who were connected with the professional field of physical education eschewed athletics in favor of milder forms of exercise for the average individual. Exercise was seen as vital for health and a major contribution to proper development, mental and moral as well as physical.

Numerous early members of the AAAPE held the medical degree, including several women. For the most part, however, their training had not included much that we would recognize today as science. To better understand their preparation and orientation, one must recall (a) the type of didactic medical training that was available to most American physicians prior to 1906, and (b) the conjunctions that were repeatedly drawn among health, exercise, and neuromuscular development, both in a biological and in a social and Darwinistic sense.

The nature of the training of most doctors who became members of the AAAPE was a significant factor in shaping the direction that the profession would take in the 20th century. Most, like Sargent—who was almost certainly more entrepreneurial than professional—had been trained according to the older didactic medical education, which was increasingly criticized for its lack of sound grounding in experimental or even clinical science. A few early AAAPE members—men like Beyer, who received both the PhD and the MD from Johns Hopkins, and Edward M. Harwell, who received the PhD in biology from Johns Hopkins in 1881 and the medical degree from Cincinnati's Miami Medical College—had extensive scientific training. So did Fitz, whose MD from Harvard had been taken under reforms that President Charles William Eliot and Henry Pickering Bowditch, MD, had instituted in the 1870s and 1880s.

It is significant that Beyer, Hartwell, and Fitz all abandoned the professional field of physical education around the turn of the century. In so doing, they left its destiny to the far less scientific, and more limited, vision of men like Sargent; to those with strong social-reform sentiments like Luther Halsey Gulick, MD, whose interests were closer to the emerging fields of social psychology and sociology; or to visionaries like Clark Hetherington. However well-intentioned his efforts, Hetherington lacked the scientific rigor of thought and technical background of men like McCurdy, McKenzie, and Thomas Denison Wood, all of whom held the MD, and all of whom, it should be noted, conceived of the field in a broad sense, drawing its rationales and research questions from disciplines ranging from physiology to philosophy.

This is not to suggest that Hetherington and others who were closer to his orientation did not have much in common with men like McCurdy and Bowen. In certain important ways they certainly did. These three, along with a significant number of substantial figures in the emerging physical education profession, were members of the Athletic Research Society, founded in 1907 to foster the scientific study of athletic problems from a national standpoint.

The orientation of this organization was toward philosophical and administrative issues. It was also, by its own declarations, deeply concerned with amateurism, and like many other contemporaries it viewed the burgeoning intercollegiate and interscholastic programs with alarm, distaste, or both. As educators first and foremost, such men perceived it their obligation (and, we must admit, in their best interests) to subscribe to what they called the amateur or the educational orientation in athletics. However, some may have been more interested in high-level elite athletics than their pronouncements suggest.

It should not be surprising that so many of the early AAAPE members took this stance; as a profession, physical education was struggling to establish itself. Even a hundred years ago there was a fairly widespread belief that professions are "based on a definable body of organized knowledge, an expertise that derives from academic training" and have, at some level, a "moral commitment of service to the public" (Hatch, 1988, pp. 1-2).

By the 1890s it had become apparent that intercollegiate athletics were more a business than anything else and that many individuals who were part of such programs lacked academic training. Either physical educators would have to take over athletic programs, which had become so entrenched that this was highly unlikely (although efforts were certainly made), or they would have to devise their own forms. To exacerbate the situation, many were exceedingly busy designing and implementing teacher training and activity programs; hence they had little time for research, even if they did have the requisite training.

The situation with regard to elite performance was compounded by the fact that a large proportion of early physical educators were women. Given Victorian and Edwardian sensibilities, they could not have been expected to demonstrate support for elite athletics. In fact, great many early female physical educators were quite aware that they were among the few females who held faculty positions in these early days. Their power was derived from those turn-of-the-century proprieties that assigned to women distinct, albeit a circumscribed, role. This gave weight to their arguments that *they* must be in charge of the physical aspects of the education of girls and women.

It was this, far more than a willingness on the part of male administrators and faculty to welcome women into their midst, that enabled distaff physical educators to establish, and in many instances dominate, their separate-sex programs. Had they even dared to opt for an athletic model, they would have put their power base in jeopardy—and they knew it. (Title IX and its consequences suggest that they were correct!)

We should return briefly to the "body of knowledge" issue. Over the last 100 years the field has vacillated from a substantially biomedical to a psychosociological, to a narrowly defined fitness, to a substantially exercise physiology/exercise science iteration of what the body of knowledge should be—all the time forgetting that since physical education deals with human beings, its roots must be in both the medical/biological and the psychosocial/cultural domains.

It is not difficult to uncover why we so often lose our way and are susceptible to passing whims and fancies. To explore this all too briefly, it will be useful to return to Fitz, the 4-year degree program at Harvard, and the extensive, if transitory, late 19th-century general interest in physical training as potentially one of the most important subjects of the curriculum. In some ways, success has been a major cause of our difficulties. The demand for teachers in the late 1800s/early 1900s was so great that a man or woman with only modest preparation might be assured of a job. McCurdy pointed to this problem in 1905 when he observed that a "man was hurried into teaching and/or coaching before he had properly prepared himself " (p. 209). Dr. Clelia Mosher (1915) made substantially the same observation to Stanford's President David Starr Jordan regarding women.

In such circumstances, 2-year normal schools, summer Chautauquas, and entrepreneurial short-duration "courses" attracted large numbers of students. Some of the best, as for example the Boston Normal School of Gymnastics (BNSG) and Sargent's Harvard Summer School, turned out quite good products. But none of these offered substantial academic/research programs, although the BNSG came reasonably close. Sargent's Harvard Summer School of Physical Training flourished, as did his entrepreneurial Sargent School of Physical Training, at the very time that Harvard's 4-year program was terminated largely for lack of students (Kroll, 1982).

Therefore, from an early date the field was decisively oriented along professional lines, with no well-organized or even adequately organized body of knowledge upon which to base its claims. It has been the absence of self-generated knowledge, not the presence of a professional paradigm, that has been our nemesis. As a consequence, we have not commanded respect from anyone and again today stand at a critical crossroads.

Since the 1960s there has been a partial reorientation of the field of physical education, broadly conceived, with considerably more attention directed at scientific and scholarly understandings of such things as the limits of human performance. (I want to make it clear that I do not limit the term science to refer to a particular methodology, but in the larger and important sense of organized and sustained pursuit of knowledge.)

True, we have tended to ignore the elite athlete, and for reasons I have tried to sketch. But what about enhancing the performance of the sedentary 60-year-old? Or the child recovering from a serious illness? What about exploring biochemical parameters and the effects of physical activity on mental functions and performance? What about seeking deeper understandings of the cultural baggage that has led to things such as anorexia, bulimia, or the recurrent fascination with shaping the body to conform to certain culturally defined ideals? And what about our responsibilities for contributing to the overall health and physical performance of the average person?

Maybe Hartwell was right when he wrote, in 1897, "Physical training has been exalted, tolerated, neglected or condemned, in varying degrees, according to the character of the conceptions concerning the nature of the human body and its relations to the human mind" (p. 357) which are extant at any period. Finding explanations for these culturally driven conceptions offers rich and still largely untilled soil for the sport historian and sport sociologist, as much if not more so than for the exercise physiologist.

If then our field is concerned with whole, integral human beings, we stand in a preeminent position to lead rather than follow. Whether this is through extending the performance of the very best athlete or through making walking a little easier for the octogenarian, our goals should probably be quite similar: (a) systematic understanding by means of carefully devised and sustained investigations of significant issues of the type that can best be generated by faculty whose aggregate proficiencies enable them to ask and address questions from multiple perspectives, and (b) intelligent and humane applications of such knowledge to all sorts of human performance.

References

Babbitt, J.A. (1901). Blood corpuscle count, haemoglobin, and sphygmograph tracing as influenced by athletic and gymnastic exercise. *American Physical Education Review*, **6**, 240-244.

Barach, J.H. (1911). Physiological and pathological effects of severe exertion (the marathon run). Physiological and pathological effects on the circulatory and renal systems. *American Physical Education Review*, **16**, 200-206.

Beyer, H.G. (1894). Football and the physique of its devotees, from the point of view of physical training. *American Journal of the Medical Sciences*, **108**, 306-322.

Bowen, W.P. (1903a). Conditions determining the rapidity of the pulse during exercise. *American Physical Education Review*, **8**, 8-15.

Bowen, W.P. (1903b). The influence of muscular work on the rate of the pulse. *American Physical Education Review*, **8**, 232-236.

Darling, E.A. (1899). The effects of training: A study of the Harvard University crew. *Boston Medical and Surgical Journal*, **141**, 229-233.

Darling, E.A. (1901). The effects of training: Second paper. *Boston Medical and Surgical Journal*, **144**, 550-559.

Fitz, G.W. (1893). Problems of physical education. *Harvard Graduates Magazine*, **2**, 26-31.

Fitz, G.W. (1895). A location reaction apparatus. *Psychological Review*, **2**, 37-42.

Flint, A. (1878). *On the source of muscular power: Arguments and conclusions upon the human subject, under conditions of rest and muscular exercise.* New York: D. Appleton & Co.

Green, H. (1986). *Fit for America: Health, fitness, sport and American society.* New York: Pantheon.

Hartwell, E.M. (1880). The study of anatomy, historically and legally considered. *Journal of Social Science*, **12**, 54-88.

Hartwell, E.M. (1897). Physical training, its function and place in education. *Boston Medical and Surgical Journal*, **137**, 357-362.

Hatch, N.O. (Ed.) (1988). *The professions in American history.* Notre Dame, IN: University of Notre Dame Press.

Hough, T. (1909). On the physiological effects of moderate muscular activity and of strain. *Science*, **29**, 484-490.

Kroll, W.P. (1982). *Graduate study and research in physical education.* Champaign, IL: Human Kinetics.

Lee, F.S. (1909). Physical exercise from the standpoint of physiology. *Science*, **29**, 521-527.

Lincoln, D.F. (1876). The nervous system as affected by schoollife. *Journal of Social Science*, **7**, 87-110.

McCurdy, J.H. (1901). The effects of maximum muscular effort on blood-pressure. *American Journal of Physiology*, **5**, 95-103.

McCurdy, J.H. (1905). A study of the characteristics of physical training in the public schools of the United States. *American Physical Education Review*, **10**, 202-213.

Mosher, C.D. (1915). [Letter to Stanford University President David Starr Jordan].

Murphy, M. (1894). *Spalding's athletic library: College athletics, training.* New York: American Sports.

Murphy, M. (1914). *Athletic training.* New York: Charles Scribner's Sons.

Peckham, G. (1887). Papers of the health department: I. The nervousness of Americans. *Journal of Social Science*, **22**, 37-49.

Putnam, J.J. (1876). Gymnastics for schools. *Journal of Social Science*, **7**, 110-124.

Sargent, D.A. (1884). Physical training in homes and training schools. *Journal of Social Science*, **18**, 44-52.

Savage, W.L. (1910). Physiological and pathological effects of severe exertion (the marathon race). *American Physical Education Review*, **15**, 651-660.

Stengel, A. (1899). The immediate and remote effects of athletics upon the heart and circulation. *American Journal of the Medical Sciences*, **118**, 544-553.

Whorton, J.C. (1982). *Crusaders for fitness: The history of American health reformers.* Princeton, NJ: Princeton University Press.

Performance Feedback and New Advances in Biomechanics

Robert J. Gregor,
Jeffrey P. Broker, and
Mimi Ryan
University of California, Los Angeles

Studying the effectiveness of various training techniques designed to improve the learning of selected motor skills is important to skill acquisition and optimization of human performance. Questions related to improved learning and long-term retention focus on the development of the most effective feedback schedule necessary for retention of a motor skill. There is a great deal of motor learning literature that addresses these issues (Adams & Reynolds, 1954; Lavery, 1962; McCracken & Stelmach, 1977; Shea & Morgan, 1979).

While the paradigms described in these reports provide a guideline for practice and feedback scheduling, many of the skills used in these studies bear little resemblance to athletic movements or performance in an athletic environment because the tasks employed are novel to the performer and relatively simple. These tasks, for example linear position or pursuit rotor tasks, usually involve discrete movements with a distinct beginning or end. In contrast, many athletic events involve continuous movement sequences without a distinct beginning or end.

Any generalizations then drawn from the data involving simple novel tasks to situations in which continuous familiar tasks are employed may require additional study. Consequently, there is a need to document the effects of various practice or feedback schedules on athletes attempting to fine-tune learned movement patterns that are part of their sport activity. This is not to imply that the need to understand simple discrete movements is unimportant but rather to say that we must expand our domain to study learning in the more complex, real-world situations.

This, in essence, is the challenge to future research efforts in the field of motor learning. To meet this challenge, I feel the tools employed and the principles and interests in the field of biomechanics may offer assistance. The merging of certain elements within each discipline has already begun in selected laboratories and should continue in the more comprehensive approach to the study of human performance.

Biomechanics

While the field of motor learning focuses on *how* we learn, the field of bio-mechanics has historically focused its research efforts on *what* variables are critical to successful performance. Scientists in the field of biomechanics seek to apply principles in engineering mechanics, mathematics, and computer science, for example, to study the function of biological systems, that is, the human body. The methods developed within this discipline, as they become more technologically sophisticated, focus in part on recording movement in a variety of settings.

The more general objective is to store, for example, visual images for sub-sequent analysis of the details of the movement pattern. This particular technique involves the use of high-speed cine film and/or standard as well as high-speed videotape systems. Once these images are properly obtained, their use and appli-cation can vary from simple feedback in the presence of the athlete and the coach to more sophisticated analyses involving complicated computer modeling.

In addition to the visual records of performance, information is obtained related to the forces generated in controlling each movement, the use of skeletal muscles important to the control of the movement, and environmental loads. Synchronization of these various pieces of information is requisite to the complete understanding of task performance.

Visual Records of Performance

High-speed film has been the traditional biomechanics research tool for the study of human movement for several decades. Specifically, in the context of this presen-tation, it has been used to provide feedback to athletes interested in analyzing their movement patterns. The advantages of using film include (a) its ability to slow the visual presentation of the movement and provide a frame by frame anal-ysis, (b) its high resolution providing the capability to monitor very small changes in position, and (c) its potential to store images for extended periods of time for repeated analysis.

The major disadvantages of 16-mm film include the cost and time required to process and print the film for subsequent analysis. For example, once the prints are made, digitizing markers placed on segment endpoints to record x,y coor-dinates of limb position on each frame of film is the most time-consuming aspect of this analysis. Although there are very sophisticated systems for analyzing film, the need to proceed frame by frame to ensure accurate recording of displacement is still very costly. This is an accurate but time-consuming method. Some of the best efforts have resulted in 24-hour turnaround of data, but there have been occasions when several months passed before the performer received information. At best, then, we do not see instantaneous feedback.

With an accurate regulation of film speed yielding a reliable time base to be used in the analysis, film provides a very precise tool for calculating velocities and accelerations. Most commonly the accelerations are used as input to equa-tions in inverse dynamics to calculate joint reaction forces, net joint moments, and net joint power. These computed variables are widely used in human move-ment analysis in musculoskeletal biomechanics and injury prevention and can be returned to athletes to inform them of performance capabilities. Again, however, computation of these outcome measures takes time, and any attempt to use these parameters as feedback will not be instantaneous.

Current efforts have focused on advancing capabilities for visual presentation by improving high-speed video technology to provide more immediate feedback for initial qualitative analyses and subsequently more detailed analyses of sport performance. These improved video systems include Super 8, standard VHS, and half-inch tape systems. While video systems are very appealing, their initial disadvantages included lack of a suitable time base for high-speed analysis and the resolution needed to measure very small changes in position.

Most current standard video systems remain at 30 to 60 Hz and cannot measure very small changes (i.e., mm) in displacement. Some of the more expensive systems, however, have higher frame rates (200 Hz or higher) and can be used quite well in research environments. Additionally, the resolution on the newer systems is improving with methods of estimating position within each pixel on the video monitor being developed. The Motion Analysis System is currently one of the more expensive systems but it does have algorithms to compute within-pixel resolution for displacement. Peak Performance is another system widely used in analysis of sport performance and it is more affordable to the consumer.

Both forms of storage systems, film and video, have been used in the laboratory under very controlled conditions as well as on the athletic field during competition. Recently, both high-speed film and high-speed video were used during world and Olympic competitions to record performances for historical purposes as well as for detailed analysis of certain events. Film records were first taken for biomechanical analysis during the 1984 Olympic Games in Los Angeles under the sponsorship of the Medical Commission of the IOC.

Recently, competitions during the Calgary Winter Olympic Games and the Seoul Summer Olympic Games were recorded using various combinations of film and video systems. Some feedback was provided to the performers within 24 hours, but most involved very time-consuming analyses that took several months to complete.

The benefit of collecting information during such elite competitions rests initially with the historical documentation of world champion athletes. Second, if appropriate arrangements are made and care is taken when data are collected, the films or videos can subsequently be analyzed to yield more precise scientific information. The major disadvantage of collecting data during such elite competitions is in the inability to completely control the data collection situation. The consequence of this lack of control is the compromise of scientific accuracy.

Regardless of some of the advantages or disadvantages of using visual images for feedback to athletes, some research teams and coaches have proceeded to use videotapes during practice to provide relatively quick qualitative feedback on some aspect of an athlete's movement pattern. This essentially is a form of summary feedback and is often used to correct certain elements identified by the coach or scientist.

The assumption in this type of analysis is that modification of a specific phase of the movement will lead to success in the total movement pattern. In baseball batting, for example, the coach may pick one part of the swing that, if improved, will lead to a better batting average. Typically the coach and athlete focus on one portion of the swing at a time, with the coach giving verbal cues and possibly a demonstration of how it should be done. With more prevalent use of video, the coach may also film several swings of the bat and have the hitter view the tapes to identify what phases of the swing need improvement.

The opportunity afforded the athlete in this case is to look at the entire performance and in a preliminary way identify certain aspects that need change. The challenge is to make sure the athlete focuses on one aspect of the movement and is not confused when several phases of the swing need work, to select a single aspect of the overall task for improvement during that training session. The human body is a linked system and what happens in one part of the system usually affects what happens in another part. These compensatory mechanisms make isolating one variable or phase of the movement quite difficult and present a challenge to the coach and athlete to set up some form of triage, making one variable critical to success and leaving other aspects of the performance to be modified later.

This example of using a discrete task in which feedback is provided on the field during practice also serves to point out the challenge of deciding which schedule is most appropriate for use in training. The athlete knows that several aspects of his swing need work. Does he select one, work on it until it has improved, and then go to the next one? Or does he try to work on two or three phases at the same time using some sophisticated schedule that in the end will result in better performance? Some ideas related to this issue and how biomechanics may be used in conjunction with motor learning will be discussed later in this paper.

A final point is that the video provides a stored image for the athletes, which may give them a greater sense of what the coach is really talking about. Often the athletes' perception of what they're doing and what actually is being done during the movement are two different things. This realization often results in the athlete attempting to recode the movement pattern and update his own internal program. This is a problem that affects the learning schedule and must be kept in mind when the retraining program begins.

On-Line Nonvisual Motion Analysis Systems

Alternatives to film and video are the active, light-emitting diode (LED) systems (e.g., Selspot & Watsmart) used primarily in the laboratory to record movement. As with the film and video, these systems can calculate 3-D coordinates from two paris of x,y coordinates acquired for two single plane cameras. Many of the motion analysis systems used currently in sports biomechanics include 3-D analysis. These 3-D coordinates are then entered into appropriate software to calculate velocities, accelerations, joint reaction forces, and net joint moments and power.

The advantage of using these LED systems is the short time delay in data reduction and analysis, although videos can be automatically scanned and digitized to derive x,y coordinate pairs of selected body markers. The major disadvantages are that (a) no visual images are recorded with the LED system, (b) they can only be used in a controlled laboratory environment, and (c) often erroneous points are stored on the computer due to reflections from the LEDs. If this type of system is used to provide feedback to athletes, it must be done in the laboratory and will only provide visual stick figures of body part movements or movements of a single point of interest to the performer and the coach.

You can use this system to provide concurrent feedback, but of a limited nature. If the limitations are not a problem (i.e., no visual image), then the system, if operating correctly, can be useful. An example of the use of this type of system will be presented later in this paper.

EMG as Biofeedback

In studying performance in the laboratory, some scientists have gone further than just using parameters related to displacement and have actually provided useful information on other performance variables. It is well documented that providing information about the electrical output of certain muscles, important to a given task, may be useful in improving performance. This form of information can be used to describe the timing sequence of muscles and can be displayed to the athlete on a computer monitor while he or she is performing the task.

Some tasks are more suitable than others to this type of feedback, but certainly this procedure has merit if used correctly. For example, scientists have placed electrodes on certain muscles in the arm and trunk during performance of the baseball pitch. This information was transmitted to a recording system and the timing of the muscles during each throw was provided to the athlete almost immediately after the pitch. This feedback was useful in determining potential problems in the throwing movement.

The challenge of course is to properly use such information during relearning or retraining of the athlete to further improve his or her movement. This type of feedback could also be done on the field with telemetry systems now being used for such purposes. Whether on the practice field or in the laboratory, however, the challenge is still the same. How is this information best used if problems are discovered and relearning or modification of the existing pattern is warranted? This information is complex and must be handled with care.

It is truly a giant step to recommend a change in patterning, especially given the large variability observed between subjects in muscle activation patterns when performing the same task. If studied correctly, however, information about EMG patterns can be useful when applied to the development of a training program involving muscles dedicated to the enhancement of the performance of a selected skill.

An example of the variability observed in the same muscle between subjects performing the same task was presented by Ryan, Gregor, and Hodgson (1988) for cycling. It seems that the biceps femoris muscle showed at least two different patterns among 25 elite cyclists performing at the same power output on a road racing bike. The point to consider here is that the same pattern may not be correct for all performers.

If we give an athlete feedback regarding muscle activity patterns and recommend that he or she follow a certain pattern demonstrated by a larger population of athletes performing the same task, we stand the risk of changing a pattern that may actually be correct for that performer. Whether the feedback is immediate, concurrent, or delayed by some period of time during which we process the EMG and make its presentation more suitable, we must be very careful about our suggestions for change.

A more appropriate procedure may be to collect this information on a performer while he or she is successful and again when there are problems. The performer then serves as his or her own standard, which minimizes erroneous change. His or her normal pattern would serve as a template for future reference and for use in future feedback training to retrain a muscle during some rehabilitation period.

Kinetic Outcome Measures

With displacements, velocities, and accelerations taken from film or video being the major source of feedback to performers, there has also been considerable effort to provide kinetic information to athletes as it relates to certain aspects of their performance. Force platforms have been used in biomechanics laboratories for many years to obtain information regarding ground reaction forces during various movements. Recently force platforms have been used in the competitive environment to provide information in a variety of sports.

Combining these data with other forms of information taken from video, film, or electromyography has become quite common, with the primary challenge being synchronization of all pieces of information. As with other forms of feedback, however, too much information could be detrimental to performance. The challenge continues to be, which variables are most important to performance enhancement?

Many people think that if they could only collect more information they would have the answer to what makes an athlete successful. Providing more information does not always improve performance; at times it may confuse the situation, especially if the information results in no clear solution to the problem.

There are many examples of ground reaction forces being shown to performers in an effort to understand, for example, running mechanics. For the past 15 years these data, including pressure patterns, have been reported in the literature and have become quite useful in identifying certain problems either with foot function per se or foot function related to certain types of running shoes. More recently, information regarding the use of force platforms in weight lifting has become more prevalent.

The study reported by Baumann, Gross, Quade, Galbierz, and Schwirtz (1988) is a good example in which force platforms were used during competition for elite athletes. The feedback to the performers was by no means instantaneous but rather was arrived at in a summary format some months later, included in a much larger analysis of weightlifting performance. Force platforms have been used in training sessions, however, and can be useful in identifying certain aspects of lifting technique.

The UCLA Biomechanics Lab has used force platforms to provide information to shot and discus throwers. Again, feedback was in a summary format since once the throwers performed a certain technique in the shotput (e.g., spin or glide) they would view their records on a computer monitor and receive some useful information for improving their performance. This last example is a classic one in which the type of information presented requires a knowledgeable individual to explain it to the athlete. If athletes were to take this information away by themselves, they may not have the understanding of what the data represent and how it relates to their performance. Consequently, information of this type, when given back to athletes, must be related to their performance or no learning will take place.

The final example in which reaction force information given to athletes may prove useful is in the sport of cycling. The UCLA Biomechanics Lab as well as those at Penn State University and the University of California, Davis, have all used some form of force pedal to provide information about lower extremity kinetics during cycling. The information is useful, of course, lending input to inverse dynamics for calculating lower extremity kinetics.

The issue that is relevant here, however, is the utility of presenting certain aspects of these reaction forces to athletes according to some feedback schedule that might actually enhance their pedaling technique and overall cycling performance. There are examples of this form of intervention in the literature in that information was presented to athletes about components of the pedal reaction force and/or pedaling angle with retention measured to evaluate learning (Gregor, Broker, & Ryan, 1991). The Biomechanics Lab at Penn State and the UCLA Human Biomechanics Lab has performed such experiments.

In summary, the field of biomechanics and the research tools used within this discipline appear to focus on the following major objectives:

1. To document loading imposed by the environment on the human body
2. To evaluate the individual response to these loads with specific reference to biological tissues in their response to load and training
3. To select variables that are important to the task and to improve these particular outcome measures to that the entire performance may be enhanced
4. To carefully consider optimization of performance and develop a suitable model for studying human performance

The important questions, then, focus on which variables are controlled to maximize performance and minimize injury.

Optimization

The last point listed above is one in which a great deal of scientific energy is now being devoted. The issue is that biomechanics as a discipline has been interested in movement analysis and in the search for a criterion variable that, if correctly modified, would optimize performance. The methods employed in optimization techniques have improved to the point that model outcomes may be given using concurrent and instant feedback to athletes so that they may improve certain elements in their performance. The assumption is that the variables under study during these feedback sessions will lead to performance optimization and may minimize injury.

As biomechanists, we have been developing faster systems of increasing complexity in order to provide this information as quickly as possible, and we have also been trying to find what selected variable we feel is highly correlated to successful performance. My point is that while we have been so interested in *what* we should provide to the athlete, the issue of *how* information should be provided was left unstudied. *What* we provide at this time is important, but *how* we provide it may be even more important to one's performance enhancement.

Even if we knew the precise variable to be modified, to be learned and incorporated into the skill pattern that would result in optimal performance, we are still faced with the problem of choosing the best method of returning information to the performer so that he or she will learn and incorporate the modifications in his or her skill pattern. Optimization techniques may provide useful information on selected variables, but if we are to effect learning then we must pay more attention to the learning schedule.

Further Comments

Certain aspects of research in biomechanics and motor control must be united. Scientists in the field of motor control who study learning should continue to expand their domain to the more complex, real-world situations and test their models using discrete tasks performed in the laboratory on these more complex outcomes. The field of biomechanics provides the utility for this expansion as well as the interest in performance enhancement and selection of criterion variables for learning. A synthesis of our methods and objectives into new approaches designed to enhance learning, and subsequently performance, is needed.

Motor Learning

The discipline of motor learning focuses on how one learns a particular task. Scientists in this field are of course interested in what variables are critical to performance, but their major concern is learning, and providing an adequate environment with suitable feedback so that one might learn in an optimal way. The disciplines of biomechanics and motor learning have been collaborating for some time, but there is a need for new energy and new collaborations between the two disciplines so that we may more completely understand which variables are more important to performance and how one might code them into his or her motor program so that injuries are minimized and performance is maximized.

The *how* portion of these motor learning experiments have typically focused on audio signals, visual signals, or other sensory signals such as touch to provide information to the athlete. Much of the testing has been done in the laboratory using novel tasks in order to understand the learning process and isolate it from the more common tasks performed every day. It is important to scientists in motor learning that novel tasks be used in order to control practice.

This is not the case, however, when dealing with elite athletes, since they face practice schedules almost every day. Additionally, the scheduling of information, whether it be immediate, summary, average, concurrent, faded, random, or blocked, must be explored with respect to an elite athlete population. Consequently, both disciplines have some common ground that needs to be cultivated.

Motor Learning/Biomechanics: Examples

Javelin

In javelin throwing, athletes seek to maximize the distance thrown. To achieve this goal, an athlete should combine movement phases in an optimal manner. Although it is difficult to identify this optimal pattern, it is just this proper sequencing that coaches and sport biomechanists look for. The javelin throw is usually divided into several phases: The initial *approach* phase usually consists of a preliminary run of 10–12 steps, which is immediately followed by a period during which the thrower makes a *transition* phase of 3–7 steps from a straight run-up approach to the final foot plant (Hay, 1985). The *release* phase is defined as the period from final right foot contact (for right-handed throwers) until javelin release. The summary effect of these three phases determines the javelin's release parameters, or initial conditions of flight, which uniquely determines the range of the implement (javelin).

In order to determine which variable is critical to a successful throw, recent research in biomechanics has focused on the flight phase, with particular emphasis on aerodynamics and the initial conditions of flight (Bartlett & Best, 1988; Hubbard & Alaways, 1987) and on the release parameters (Gregor & Pink, 1985; Whiting, Gregor, & Halushka, 1991). Since proper segment orientation and movement sequencing play a central role in determining the success of a throw, the study by Whiting et al. (1991) examined the contributions made by different body segments to the success of throws in a large population of elite athletes. Eight male javelin throwers were filmed while throwing new-rules javelins during competition at five meets over a 2-year period. Body segment kinematics and javelin release parameters were assessed relative to their contribution to throwing performance.

The data suggest that successful throws, as judged by distance thrown, are characterized by higher release speeds, longer last-step lengths, less flexion of the front leg knee during the final plant phase, and an orderly progression of peak speeds at the hip, shoulder, and elbow from the onset of double leg support until release. Individual variability in performance was associated with differences measured between several throwing variables.

While the data in this study suggest several trends characteristic of successful throwing, there is a lack of significance in comparing many of the measures to distance thrown. More detailed investigation revealed that many differences appear specific to the individual throwers. This observation is consistent with previous literature in which Hubbard and Alaways (1987) caution against reliance on globally optimized regression equations, noting that they be interpreted with care.

Although certain general findings (such as the beneficial effect of a high release speed) may be applicable to all throwers, careful individual assessment is required, especially at the elite level, if optimal performance is to be attained. This is due to the complexity of this particular event and to the sensitivity of the final result to the many variables affecting throwing distance.

While Whiting et al. (1991) showed considerable variability in parameters related to javelin release in an elite group of throwers, Hubbard and Alaways (1987) concentrated on feedback during practice sessions in an effort to present selected aspects of the flight of the javelin immediately after release that may be useful in improving the thrower's performance. They developed a system to measure five release conditions, which were presented to the thrower in a summary feedback format within minutes after the throw.

A 2-D motion analysis system was used to collect video images of the javelin for the first 0.1 to 0.2 seconds after release and to automatically digitize (200 Hz) x,y position data of selected marker points on the javelin. The system then estimated five release conditions from the x,y coordinate data and graphically presented them to the thrower together with a simulation of the subsequent flight. These data were also compared to optimal release and flight conditions using the same release velocity and nonlinear optimization algorithms.

The unique aspect of this study is that it represents the first reported attempt to critique, nearly instantly in a precise quantitative manner, the critical factors in the throw that determine the range of the javelin. Identification of crucial factors at release are a bit easier than determining thrower techniques that will lead to improved performance, and Hubbard and Alaways have gone a step further and actually considered the method of feedback. No mention was made of concerns over scheduling, but that is the next step.

Running

With improvement in technology and the use of laboratory facilities that can be expanded to include a simulation of the performance environment, some scientists have begun to use more immediate forms of feedback to guide the performer into modifying selected performance variables. The assumption again is that the selected variable is most important to that task and is one that warrants all their attention.

Keith Williams at the University of California, Davis, has provided kinematic feedback to runners on the treadmill. In his study of distance runners and the collection of data on elite distance runners, Williams found that the knee angle during the recovery phase was an important element in running style. Some of his data actually indicated that certain ranges of knee angles may enhance performance during the swing phase of running. He would provide this information to the athlete and coach or teach them to concentrate on keeping the knee angle in a certain range.

Additionally, Peter Cavanagh at Penn State University has provided information to runners on a treadmill that tells them something about vertical movement of the body. It has been well documented in the physiology and biomechanics literature that unnecessary vertical movements of the body during running are costly and inefficient. Consequently, each runner attempts to minimize the vertical oscillation and any other extraneous movements that are not dedicated to the success of the task.

Using a Selspot System, which is essentially an active position-indicating system (LED system previously mentioned), Cavanagh would place a marker on the head of the runners and have them follow its movement on a computer monitor. This information, provided immediately to the athletes and actually concurrent with their performance, would be used as feedback in order to enhance their running performance. The obvious objective here was to minimize the vertical movement of that marker in that it would be associated with the vertical movement of the body that the runner was trying to minimize in order to enhance performance. In this particular example, the relationship between the variable selected for modification and performance success, to improve efficiency, is clearer than in other events.

Cycling

Augmented feedback was used by David Sanderson (1986) to modify the riding mechanics of inexperienced cyclists. Use of this procedure was part of Sanderson's doctoral work under the direction of Peter Cavanagh at Penn State University. An experimental and a control group practiced for 32 minutes for each of 10 days, with retention tests given immediately and 7 days after the acquisition period was completed. All subjects were instructed to reduce the force applied to the pedal during a small region of the recovery phase (225 to 315° after top dead center).

While both groups received information about cadence, only the experimental group received visual feedback. This feedback represented the computed average of the left and right leg resultant force impulses on the pedal, averaged over five consecutive pedaling cycles and presented every seventh revolution. The feedback schedule was modified during acquisition such that the time with and without feedback varied from 50:50 initially to 10:90 in the last days.

Following this protocol, the experimental group was able to reduce the force impulse during the recovery phase (180°–360°) to the values seen at the end of acquisition during the first day of practice. The control group was able to reduce the force impulse at the pedal but not to the extent attained by the experimental group. The retention tests indicated that the experimental group was able to maintain the same level of proficiency as at the end of acquisition.

These results indicated that force application during the cycling task can be modified using augmented visual feedback. The feedback schedule (averaged and faded) used by Sanderson has proven very effective in a number of motor learning experiments using simple skills. Sanderson's results indicate that the motor learning paradigms for simple skills may generalize to more complex tasks. This study also supports the need to continue using such techniques in biomechanics in conjunction with motor learning theory to improve performance. The potential benefits of this combination are obvious.

Although several investigators have recently reported successful modification of bicycle pedaling technique using real-time or concurrent biomechanical feedback, the extent to which the practiced pedaling patterns represent permanent or learned capabilities is questionable.

Recent data suggest that frequent feedback can interfere with learning by promoting learner dependency on the feedback. Broker and Gregor (1989) evaluated the retention of a cycling kinetic pattern using two different feedback schedules, and evaluated the potential for feedback dependency in a continuous task learning environment. Eighteen inexperienced cyclists rode a racing bicycle mounted to a fixed-fork Velodyne trainer at 125 W (78 rpm). Pedal forces were monitored by dual piezoelectric transducers within each pedal (Broker & Gregor, 1990).

Subjects were assigned to concurrent (CFB) or summary (SFB) feedback groups and performed 50 one-minute practice trials, receiving right-pedal shear force feedback and a criterion pattern emphasizing effective shear near 0 and 180° in the pedaling cycle. CFB subjects received concurrent feedback 140 ms after completing every other revolution while SFB subjects received averaged feedback between trials. All subjects performed 10 retention trials without feedback 1 week later.

Both groups improved significantly during practice. Performance decay in retention was negligible for both groups. Group differences during all phases were not significant. High CFB group proficiency in retention indicated that the detrimental aspects of frequent feedback were not significant in this task. High SFB proficiency in retention suggests that large changes in kinetic patterning are achievable with relatively few feedback presentations.

Current interests in the use of feedback to enhance performance focus on whether random or blocked feedback scheduling is the most effective for learning several components of one task. Using the cycling task, an initial objective of current studies at UCLA is to establish whether feedback regarding different aspects of the cycling task are learned more effectively with a random or a blocked feedback schedule.

In the last decade, motor learning experiments have refuted the view that blocked practice is better for learning than random practice of the same tasks (Lee & Magill, 1983; Salmoni, Schmidt, & Walter, 1984; Shea & Morgan, 1979). This paradigm involves a blocked group that practices one task until it is perfected before learning the next task component. The random group involves learning the same tasks but in a random order. This research shows that the random condition is more effective for learning than the blocked condition, as measured by long-term retention.

A theory underlying these findings is that the random condition forces the learner to process the feedback information at a deeper and more meaningful level than the blocked condition. More distinctions between the feedback given for each task are made by the random group, enhancing the learning of the various tasks. Another explanation is that in the random condition the learner forgets the solution to performing the task, whereas the blocked condition allows the learner to remember the solution.

Because the random group must later recall the solution, the learner practices retrieving the appropriate information to perform the task, which is what he or she will have to do when no feedback is given. The random group therefore will learn more effectively than the blocked group because the former is able to develop or learn association between the different task variations and is also forced to retrieve the information from long-term memory.

These data all involved variations of a task while keeping feedback type and schedule constant. One might hypothesize that subjects could be encouraged to utilize the same processes (intertrial associations and retrieval practice) if the task were held constant with the feedback schedule being manipulated. This type of analysis can be tested in both discrete and continuous tasks; however, the use of a continuous task such as cycling could provide unique and interesting information. This manipulation would allow the blocked versus random paradigm to be applied to the feedback schedule as opposed to the task schedule. By receiving feedback about different components of the same task (random schedule), the learner would be encouraged to practice retrieval and intertrial associations.

Another manipulation that must be considered is *when* the feedback should be given. Either immediate or summary feedback can be used, with many individuals advocating immediate feedback as the most beneficial. However, data on discrete tasks indicate that summary feedback is better for learning and long-term retention of skills. Summary feedback is provided to the subject after a specific set of trials has been completed. The feedback is a simultaneous presentation of all trials in the previous trial set.

The generalization to continuous tasks has not been widely studied; however, this was explored in a study at UCLA (Broker & Gregor, 1990). Data from that study indicate that immediate feedback was no worse than summary feedback for learning. Summary feedback appeared to be as good as if not better than immediate feedback, and easier to process and present when compared to immediate feedback.

After a feedback protocol (random or blocked) has been established as being the most effective for learning, one may then propose certain techniques that will improve the pedaling techniques of selected junior or senior elite riders. Working with the cycling coaches will be vitally important in establishing the technique parameters that need modification as specified for each rider.

One final aspect that should be studied when using the cycling task is how the legs (right side vs. left side) interact to perform the task. Data by Broker and Gregor (1990) indicate that feedback given about the dominant leg did not aid in transfer of learning to the nondominant leg. In that study, however, subjects were not instructed to have symmetry between the legs. In future studies the subjects may be instructed to be symmetrical. It is important therefore to determine whether feedback about the dominant leg will transfer to the nondominant leg and/or whether feedback about the nondominant leg will transfer to the dominant leg.

Summary

While we have discussed many examples of how scientists have combined interests in biomechanics and motor learning, the need to continue these efforts is obvious. The motor learning tasks must become better related to actual sport events, and the scientists in biomechanics must be more aware of the manner in which information about the many variables under study is conveyed to the athletes. There is a common ground to combine the *what* with the *how* and apply our common knowledges to more complex tasks.

References

Adams, J.A., & Reynolds, B. (1954). Effect of shift and distribution of practice conditions following interpolated rest. *Journal of Experimental Psychology*, **47**, 32-36.

Bartlett, R.M., & Best, R.J. (1988). The biomechanics of javelin throwing: A review. *Journal of Sports Sciences*, **6**, 1-38.

Baumann, W., Gross, V., Quade, K., Galbierz, P., & Schwirtz, A. (1988). The snatch technique of world class weightlifters at the 1985 world weightlifting championships. *International Journal of Sport Biomechanics*, **4**, 68-89.

Broker, J.P., & Gregor, R.J. (1989). Extrinsic feedback and the learning of cycling kinetic patterns. *Journal of Biomechanics*, **22**, 991.

Broker, J.P., & Gregor, R.J. (1990). A dual piezoelectric element force pedal for kinetic analysis of cycling. *International Journal of Sport Biomechanics*, **6**, 394-404.

Gregor, R.J., Broker, J.P., Ryan, M.M. (1991). Biomechanics of cycling. In John Halloszy (Ed.), *Exercise and sports sciences reviews* (Vol. 19, pp. 127-169). Philadelphia: Williams & Wilkens.

Gregor, R.J., & Pink, M. (1985). Biomechanical analysis of a world record javelin throw: A case study. *International Journal of Sport Biomechanics*, **1**, 73-77.

Hay, J.G. (1985). *The biomechanics of sports techniques*. New York: Prentice Hall.

Hubbard, M., & Alaways, L.W. (1987). Optimum release conditions for the new-rules javelin. *International Journal of Sport Biomechanics*, **3**, 207-221.

Lavery, J.J. (1962). Retention of simple motor skills as a function of type of knowledge of results. *Canadian Journal of Psychology*, **16**, 300-311.

Lee, T.D., & Magill, R.A. (1983). The locus of contextual interference and motor skill acquisition. *Journal of Experimental Psychology: Learning, Memory and Cognition*, **9**, 730-746.

McCracken, H.D., & Stelmach, G.E. (1977). A test of the schema theory of discrete motor learning. *Journal of Motor Behavior*, **9**, 193-201.

Ryan, M., Gregor, R.J., & Hodgson, J.A. (1988). Neural patterning of lower extremity muscles during cycling at a constant load. *Journal of Biomechanics*, **21**, 854.

Salmoni, A.W., Schmidt, R.A., & Walter, C.B. (1984). Knowledge of results and motor learning: A review and critical reappraisal. *Psychological Bulletin*, **95**, 355-386.

Sanderson, D.J. (1986). An application of a computer based real-time data acquisition and feedback system. *International Journal of Sport Biomechanics*, **2**, 210-214.

Shapiro, D., Zernicke, R.F., Gregor, R.J., & Diestel, J.D. (1981). Evidence for generalized motor programs using gait pattern analysis. *Journal of Motor Behavior*, **13**, 33-47.

Shea, J.B., & Morgan, R.L. (1979). Contextual interference effects on the acquisition, retention and transfer of motor skill. *Journal of Experimental Psychology: Human Learning and Memory*, **5**, 179-187.

Whiting, W.C., Gregor, R.J., & Halushka, M. (1991). Kinematic analysis of body segment and release parameter contributions to new-rules javelin throwing by experienced male throwers. *International Journal of Sport Biomechanics*, **7**, 111-124.

Reaction to Performance Feedback: Advances in Biomechanics

James G. Hay
The University of Iowa

In reacting to the paper by Dr. Gregor, I propose first to address some of the issues he has raised, and second, to raise an additional question concerning the role of biomechanists in enhancing the performance of elite athletes.

Service and Research Functions

Most biomechanists working to enhance performance in sport do so in one or two ways. Some analyze the performance of specific athletes and provide information to their coaches with the express intent of assisting them in their efforts to improve the athletes' performance. They thus perform a *service, or clinical* function. They take existing technology, procedures, and knowledge and apply them to the benefit of the performer. Instead, or in addition, some biomechanists perform a *research* function. They seek to extend our knowledge of sports techniques and injury mechanisms and to develop improved sporting apparel and equipment.

Under the best of circumstances these two roles go hand in hand. In the course of performing a service role, the biomechanist identifies the major technical issues in the sport concerned. He or she then formulates appropriate research questions and pursues them to their logical conclusion. When the results of this research suggest changes in current coaching practices, as is often the case, the biomechanist, once again operating in a service mode, incorporates these changes in his or her analyses and subsequent recommendations.

Although the UCLA work described by Dr. Gregor may or may not have had its genesis in service work on cycling, it is a good example of the "return journey"—the research-to-practice part of this desirable circular relationship between the service and research components of such work.

New Technologies

Dr. Gregor referred to the increasing use of videography as a replacement for 16-mm cinematography in analyses of human motion. The development of videography has had a profound effect in recent years on the study of the techniques used in sports. Videotape is much cheaper to use than 16-mm film. In 1988 we spent $2,000 for the film and processing required to record three long and triple jump events at the U.S. Olympic Trials; in 1989 we spent just $62 for videotapes to record performances in the same events at the national championships. The processing of videotape is much quicker. In 1988 it took 3 weeks to have our 16-mm film shipped, processed, and returned; in 1989 the processing was done instantaneously. The videotape was available for viewing immediately after the recording stopped.

The cost of basic S-VHS camcorders, digitizing systems, and associated software is roughly comparable to the corresponding 16-mm items. However, there is one major limitation: high-speed video cameras are still about twice the price of high-speed, 16-mm film cameras. Hopefully, a growing demand and increased competition will soon eliminate this problem.

It is perhaps of some interest to note here that, apart from the increasing use of three-dimensional techniques, which are rapidly replacing the traditional two-dimensional ones, improvements in technology and methodology have had relatively little impact on the procedures used to gather and analyze biomechanical data on competitive sports performances.

Force platforms have occasionally been installed in strategic positions at major events to obtain kinetic data on the techniques used, as for example at the 1985 world weightlifting championships in Sweden (Baumann, Gross, Quade, Galbierz, & Ansgar, 1988) and at the 1986 world diving championships in Spain (Miller, Hennig, Pizzimenti, Jones, & Nelson, 1989; Miller, Jones, Pizzimenti, Hennig, & Nelson, 1990). But the sophisticated opto-electronic and video-based automatic digitizing systems that have had a pronounced impact on the study of human walking, and on other activities for which appropriate data can be obtained under controlled laboratory conditions, have not yet to the best of my knowledge been used under the competitive conditions of elite sport.

Monitoring Versus Analyzing

Dr. Gregor raised an issue on which almost all elite athletes, their coaches, and the sport scientists with whom they work seem to agree—the importance of prompt feedback. The argument most often advanced in support of prompt feedback is that information on the technique an athlete used days, weeks, or months ago is of little value because his or her technique may change with time. What is needed instead, it is said, is an evaluation of the athlete's technique *today*.

In my view, discussion on this point is often confused because those who argue for immediate feedback do not draw what I believe to be a critical distinction, the distinction between analyzing and monitoring the athlete's technique.

Analyzing an athlete's technique is a comprehensive, theory-based process designed to identify the biomechanical factors that distinguish good performances from lesser performances for that athlete. It involves painstaking data collection, reduction, and processing. It also involves a thorough and thoughtful evaluation of the results and an interpretation of what they mean in the practical context.

Given appropriate facilities, equipment, and personnel, the time needed to perform the data collection, reduction, and processing steps can be reduced to a bare minimum. The time needed to interpret the results should not, in my view, be similarly reduced to a minimum. To do so increases the risk of misinterpreting the data and misleading the athlete and coach. We must be very careful not to take thinking out of the process of analyzing the techniques of elite athletes!

When I am pressed by a coach or an athlete for the results of an analysis, I usually respond by asking gently, "How would you like this analysis done? Quickly or correctly?" Naturally they want both, but if they must choose—and of course they must—they usually recognize that the immediacy of the feedback is much less important than its validity.

Monitoring the technique of an athlete is something quite different from all of this. It usually involves the determination of a number of characteristics of an athlete's technique that have been found relevant to his or her success. For example, Mont Hubbard of the University of California, Davis, has developed a sophisticated system for use in the training of javelin throwers. This automated, opto-electronic system yields data on such variables as the speed and angle of release, the attitude angle, and the angle of attack immediately after the throw is completed.

There is an obvious and important place in athletics for such systems. They are especially useful in monitoring how an athlete is progressing from trial to trial in his or her efforts to make a change in technique. However, they are not systems for the comprehensive analysis of techniques. To expect immediate feedback from a system designed to monitor the progress of an athlete is only right and proper. To expect immediate feedback from a comprehensive biomechanical analysis is folly.

Feedback Scheduling

Dr. Gregor has raised some intriguing issues concerning the form of the feedback provided to an athlete, and it will be very interesting to see whether the findings from controlled laboratory studies of movements with little similarity to those found in athletics are also true of the leg movements seen in cycling. These movements, I might add, are themselves about as constrained as athletic movements ever get.

Dr. Gregor described a basic two-step procedure. In the first step, the technique variables to be modified are identified. He called this the "what" part of the process; I'd call it the analysis part. In the second step, some form of feedback is given with a view to improving the athlete's performance by modifying one or more of these technique variables. The effectiveness of this "how" part of the process, as he has called it, is carefully monitored using special bicycle pedals instrumented to yield measures of the forces exerted by the athlete.

The first of these two steps, involving a biomechanical analysis of leg motions in cycling, clearly falls within the domain or area of expertise of the sport biomechanist. The second, involving the use of force-measuring and perhaps other equipment to evaluate learning schedules, just as clearly falls within what I will call motor learning.

Biomechanics and motor learning, behavior and control have much in common, and it is no surprise therefore that those whose area of specialization is biomechanics address issues that would normally be considered to lie in one of these other areas. We at Iowa, for example, have conducted studies on the use of visual control during the final strides of the approach in the long jump, triple jump, and pole vault, and on how to improve an athlete's ability to use visual control to bring him or her accurately to the point of takeoff.

I'm not really sure what I think about such departures from one's area of expertise. Obviously, if you have a passionate interest in a research question and the path to an answer passes into areas outside your expertise, you either recruit experts and assemble a multidisciplinary team or you acquire the needed knowledge yourself by whatever means you have at your disposal. In such cases, the question is clearly paramount and whatever price it exacts must be paid. In other cases, perhaps like the present one described by Dr. Gregor, the problem may be that the results of research conducted in one field cannot be applied effectively in practice because the necessary research has yet to be conducted in some adjoining field.

Here the issue is much less clear, at least in my mind. Should you move into the development part of what industry refers to as research and development and "get the product to the marketplace"? Or should you return to what you're best at and get on with the next project, leaving the development of your research findings to take its natural course?

Contribution of Sport Biomechanics

Although a few sport biomechanists were already providing scientific services to elite athletes and their coaches, it was the initiation of the Elite Athlete Project by the U.S. Olympic Committee in 1982 that provided the main impetus for the present level of service and research activity. Thus there has been some 8 to 9 years in which such activity has been pursued with varying degrees of vigor in this country.

During this time, sport biomechanists have worked hard to develop procedures for analyzing the performances of athletes and conveying information to coaches and athletes that may be of use to them in their preparations for major competitions. The biomechanists have also been working continually to improve the procedures they use, with a view to increasing the value of the assistance they offer.

Thus, for example, we started in 1982 using a high-speed motion picture camera to record in side view the actions of our top long jumpers during the last four strides of the approach and the takeoff, and another to record their actions during the takeoff, flight, and landing. We then conducted two-dimensional analyses of the resulting film records and prepared a simple report with our results and recommendations to coaches and athletes.

Today we use one panning videocamera to record the athlete's actions from the start of the approach to the landing in the sand, and two other panning videocameras to record the athlete's motions during the last four strides, the takeoff, flight, and landing. We then take the videotape from the first camera, analyze the athlete's performance during the approach, and run the data with an expert system that performs the necessary computations, evaluates the results against established norms, and prints a report containing recommended training drills and other suggestions for improvement.

The videotapes from the other two cameras are analyzed to provide a three-dimensional analysis of the athlete's performance during the transition from approach to takeoff and during the jump itself. The resulting report contains three-dimensional graphics showing the athlete's performance in top, side, and rear views, together with more complete detail than ever offered in any analysis of the event.

During this same period, from 1982 to the present, the most often-asked question about the Elite Athlete Project and its various successors has been, "What effect has it had on the performances of American athletes?" And the entirely unsatisfactory but truthful answer is, "No one knows."

Because of the many factors that have an influence on an athlete's performance for good or ill, and because it is virtually impossible to measure these separate influences, there is no way to gauge with confidence the effect that our efforts have had. Over this period we have greatly increased the number of athletes and coaches for whom we provide services. We have greatly increased the scope and sophistication of our services. We have gained a great deal of experience and knowledge of the motor skills involved. We have increased the number and extent of our interactions with coaches and athletes.

But, at the end of the day, as the British are fond of saying, we still cannot prove we are having any effect at all. Our athletes are still winning gold medals and breaking world records, so it is clear that we are not doing irreparable harm. But beyond that we are unable to go with much confidence.

This is a serious obstacle. It prevents us from evaluating the effectiveness of what we are doing because we have no reliable criterion upon which to base such evaluation. It limits our effectiveness in the political and especially in the funding arenas because we have nothing to show for our efforts that provides compelling evidence for continued or enhanced funding.

Under these circumstances we are obliged to do the best we can on the basis of the anecdotal accounts and reactions of the coaches, athletes, and administrators with whom we work. We must rely on the occasional public, and more frequently the private, statements of coaches and athletes about the benefits they believe they have derived from our efforts.

Finally, and most frustrating of all, it is not a problem that shows any prospect of solution, nor is it one that is likely to go away.

References

Baumann, W., Gross, V., Quade, K., Galbierz, P., & Ansgar, S. (1988). The snatch technique of world class weightlifters at the 1985 World Championships. *International Journal of Sport Biomechanics*, **4**, 68-89.

Miller, D.I., Hennig, E., Pizzimenti, M.A., Jones, I.C., & Nelson, R.C. (1989). Kinetic and kinematic characteristics of 10-m platform performances of elite divers: I. Back takeoffs. *International Journal of Sport Biomechanics*, **5**, 60-88.

Miller, D.I., Jones, I.C., Pizzimenti, M.A., Hennig, E., & Nelson, R.C. (1990). Kinetic and kinematic characteristics of 10-m platform performances of elite divers: II. Reverse takeoffs. *International Journal of Sport Biomechanics*, **6**, 283-308.

Practice Schedule Considerations for Enhancing Human Performance in Sport

Richard A. Magill
Louisiana State University

The preparation of athletes for sport performance involves many different components. Among these is the development of effective practice regimes that will provide opportunities for the athlete to prepare his or her skill so that its performance will be optimal during competition. Included in the several considerations related to developing effective practice regimes is the organization of schedules for the practice periods that must be planned prior to competition. All of the skills to be learned or improved must not only be incorporated into these schedules but also organized in a way that will provide the most effective preparation possible.

It is this organizational aspect of developing practice schedules that is the focus of this paper. The view presented here is that, for certain skills, there are practice schedule organization schemes that lead to better preparation than others. The aim of this discussion is to establish what the motor learning research literature indicates concerning which practice schedule organizations provide optimal preparation for enhancing performance for different sport skills.

Practice—Test Relationship Concerns

Before discussing practice schedule organization, there must be an understanding of an important principle that directly relates to this issue. When interest is directed toward determining the effectiveness of a practice related variable, it is essential that the effectiveness of the practice variable be determined only on the basis of performance during the competition rather than during the practice sessions.

This principle has been promoted as an important characteristic of learning research for at least half a century but has been ignored at various times in the research literature (e.g., Adams, 1987; Tolman, 1932). However, the importance of this principle has been reestablished in recent years (see Magill, 1989; Schmidt, 1988), as empirical evidence has shown that inferences about the effectiveness for learning various practice variables can be misleading when they are based on practice performance rather than on test performance.

An excellent example can be seen in the review of knowledge of results (KR) research published by Salmoni, Schmidt, and Walter (1984). They effectively demonstrated that certain "laws" of KR hold for performance only during practice trials but not for performance on retention or transfer tests given at some later time.

In some instances, performance that was better during practice under the influence of one level of a particular variable was not different from other levels of that variable on the retention or transfer test. In other cases, the performance on the test was worse than performance under the influence of another level of that variable. Since the focus of enhancing sport performance must be the preparation for an upcoming test, it is essential that test performance be the basis for determining the effectiveness of practice variables and not practice performance.

Contextual Interference as a Practice Schedule Phenomenon

In the study of motor skill learning, a learning phenomenon that relates directly to the issue of organizing practice schedules is known as the contextual interference effect. This effect is related to practice situations in which several variations of a skill must be learned or prepared. There are many examples of this in motor skills, as indicated by the following few situations: A tennis player must learn several types of serves. A baseball batter must be prepared to hit several types of pitches. A child must learn to throw an object using different throwing patterns. And a dancer must often learn several variations of a dance sequence.

The contextual interference effect indicates that when certain skill variations are practiced in preparation for an upcoming test, high levels of "interference" lead to better test performance than low levels. What is being referred to here is the interference that results from how the practice schedule is organized to enable learning the skill variations. The interference results from the arrangement of trials within the practice context itself, hence the term contextual interference.

A high level of contextual interference occurs when the skill variations are practiced in a random arrangement of trials whereas a low level results from practicing the skill variations in a blocked arrangement in which each skill variation is practiced in its own block, or unit, of trials. Thus, contextual interference should be seen as a continuum of interference where low and high are descriptors at the extremes, indicating the amount of interference.

Battig's Demonstration of the Effect.   The contextual interference effect was originally demonstrated for learning verbal skills by Battig (1966, 1972, 1979). He used contextual interference as a basis for arguing that interference does not always lead to negative transfer in learning, which was the prevailing view of interference. In the contextual interference case just the opposite occurs, as transfer test performance is benefited by increasing amounts of interference during practice.

Battig showed that low levels of contextual interference lead to better practice performance than high levels. However, during a transfer test, performance deteriorates. On the other hand, high levels of contextual interference during practice lead to improved transfer test performance. Thus, interference during practice is *beneficial* in preparing for an upcoming test.

Initial Motor Skill Demonstration.   For motor skills, the first demonstration of the contextual interference effect was reported by Shea and Morgan (1979). In their experiment, subjects were required to learn to move one arm as quickly as possible through three different three-segment patterns. In response to a stimulus light, the subject picked up a tennis ball, knocked over a series of three freely movable wooden barriers with the ball, and then returned the ball to a final location.

The three prescribed movement patterns were illustrated on cards that were visible to subjects and located above a colored stimulus light specific to that pattern. Performance was measured by total response time, which was measured as the time that elapsed between the onset of the appropriate stimulus light and placing the ball in the final location.

Contextual interference was incorporated into the practice schedule by using a blocked practice schedule, representing a low level of contextual interference, and a random schedule, representing a high level of contextual interference. In the blocked schedule, subjects practiced all 18 trials of practice for one movement pattern before practicing another pattern. The random schedule distributed the 18 trials for each movement pattern randomly among the 54 total practice trials.

It is important to note that both groups had the same amount of practice trials for each movement pattern and the same length of time between trials. The only difference between these practice conditions was the organization of the practice trials. Retention and transfer tests were administered to all subjects as tests of learning. These occurred 10 minutes and 10 days after the practice trials ended. The retention tests involved performing the three practiced movement patterns while the transfer tests involved moving through a new three-segment pattern and a five-segment pattern.

Results of this experiment supported four important predictions from Battig's discussion of the effect of contextual interference. First, the blocked practice schedule yielded better performance than the random schedule during the practice trials. Second, those who had the random practice performed better on the retention tests. Third, performance was better for subjects who had a random practice schedule but a blocked test schedule than for those who had a blocked practice schedule but a random test schedule. Fourth, the random practice condition led to better performance than the blocked practice condition on both transfer tasks.

Thus, lower levels of contextual interference lead to superior practice performance but result in poorer retention and transfer test performance than random practice. And random practice appears to have an added benefit of increasing adaptability to novel performance situations, which was shown by the results of the two transfer tests and by the retention tests wherein the performance schedules differed from what was practiced.

Establishing the Generalizability. A question that has emerged from the findings of Shea and Morgan (1979) as well as from the more theoretical accounts of these results by Shea and Zimny (1983) has concerned the generalizability of the contextual interference effect. Is it a general learning phenomenon related to practice schedule organization or is it only related to certain laboratory task learning situations? It seems clear at this point that the contextual interference effect is indeed a learning phenomenon related to more than just certain laboratory situations.

Support for the effect has been reported for several laboratory tasks as well as for nonlaboratory tasks (see Magill & Hall, 1990, for a review of this literature). Since the focus of this paper is on sport performance, an example of the contextual interference effect for learning a sport skill will illustrate how this effect has been effectively generalized to the sport domain.

An experiment reported by Goode and Magill (1986) involved university students in beginning badminton classes learning three serves: the long, short, and drive serves. One group practiced these serves by following a modified blocked schedule in which one serve was practiced for 36 trials on Monday, one on Wednesday, and one on Friday for each of 3 weeks. For another group, the three serves were randomly practiced whereby any of the three serves could be performed on each trial of these same 9 days of practice. Thus every subject practiced each serve for 108 trials, which yielded a total of 324 trials.

The most striking results were seen on the transfer test, in which all subjects were required to use these same three serves but from the left service court. All the practice trials had been from the right service court. Performance of the random practice group showed no change from the end of practice whereas the group with the blocked practice schedules performed from the new service court like they had at the beginning of their practice trials.

Thus the contextual interference effect was found for learning badminton serves and showed that higher levels of contextual interference not only benefit retention of practiced skills but also increase one's capability to adapt the learned skills to new performance situations.

Skill Characteristics and the Contextual Interference Effect

While the research investigating the contextual interference effect has shown that this effect generalizes to a variety of laboratory and sport skills, the empirical evidence has also shown that it does not generalize to every skill or learning situation. Perhaps most important for the present discussion are those limits of the effect that are related to the type of skill being learned and the individual's stage of learning.

Control by Different Versus Same Motor Programs. In their review of the research investigating the contextual interference effect, Magill and Hall (1990) proposed a hypothesis concerning skill characteristics that predict when the effect would and would not be found. They hypothesized that when the skill variations to be learned are controlled by *different* motor programs, then the contextual interference effect would be found when practice schedules were compared. However, when the skill variations to be learned are controlled by the *same* motor program, then the contextual interference effect either would not be found or it would be found only after some modification of the high versus low contextual interference practice schedule situation.

The term "motor program" in the Magill and Hall hypothesis is related to the term "generalized motor program" as described by Schmidt (1975, 1988). He argued that the generalized motor program serves as a memory representation for a movement class rather than for one movement. A movement class can be defined by its invariant characteristics. When a variety of actions have common invariant features, they are considered to be in the same movement class and controlled by the same motor program.

Several different movement characteristics have been proposed by Schmidt and by others to be the invariant features of a motor program. Some examples are relative timing, which relates to the rhythmic structure of the components of an action, relative force, and sequence of events of an action.

It is important to note that there is continuing debate concerning the validity of the generalized motor program construct and of the identity of the invariant features defining the program (see Gentner, 1987, 1988; Heuer, 1988; Heuer & Schmidt, 1988). However, the application of the generalized motor program construct to establishing skill characteristic parameters of the contextual interference effect appears appropriate, as results of research investigating this effect seem to fall into categories that are aptly defined by this motor program view. As such, the motor program construct serves as a useful heuristic for establishing why the contextual interference effect has been found in some research studies but not in others.

In the Magill and Hall (1990) hypothesis, variations of a skill were assumed to be under the control of the *same* motor program if the relative timing, sequence of events, and/or spatial configurations remained constant across the practiced skill variations. Thus, skill variations have this control characteristic require subjects to modify certain parameters of the skill in order to perform it. For example, if a person is practicing throwing a ball at a target and the goal is to learn to throw it at different speeds, then all that is needed to produce the different speeds is to modify the overall force parameter of the throwing action.

On the other hand, if the skill variations being practiced are characterized by different relative timing, relative force, sequence of events, and/or spatial configurations of the movement pattern, then the skill variations were assumed to be controlled by *different* motor programs. An example here in the ball throwing situation would be when the person must learn to throw the ball at the target using different throwing patterns, such as an overhand, underhand, and sidearm throw.

What is important here is that there is empirical evidence to support the Magill and Hall (1990) hypothesis. In contextual interference experiments, when motor skills have involved learning different movement patterns such as the barrier knockdown task used by Shea and Morgan (1979) and by others (e.g., Lee & Magill, 1983; Wood & Ging, 1991), maze tracing tasks (Jelsma & Pieters, 1989), and badminton serving (Goode & Magill, 1986), the contextual interference effect consistently has been found.

However, in experiments when the motor skill variations being practiced involved a parameter modification to produce the different variations, the contextual interference effect has not been found. Some examples of this type of learning situation include performing a three-segment barrier knockdown task in which only one pattern is performed but the goal is to move through the pattern at different specified movement times (Poto, 1988, Experiment 2), performing a multicomponent movement pattern in which the variations involve different sizes of the same pattern (Wood & Ging, 1991), and pursuit rotor tracking, wherein the pattern remains the same but tracking involves different speeds (Whitehurst & Del Rey, 1983).

An interesting feature of experiments involving parameter modifications is that the results suggest that combinations of high and low contextual interference schedules may work best for these learning situations.

An experiment by Pigott and Shapiro (1984) illustrates this point. They had children learn to throw beanbags of three different weights at a target, which is an example of learning skill variations that involve modifying the overall force parameter. What is noteworthy about the results of this experiment is that the practice condition that led to the best transfer test performance was a mixed random and blocked practice condition in which three-trial blocks of each beanbag weight were randomly scheduled.

Magill and Hall (1990) argued that the basis for the different results for skill variations being controlled by different motor programs versus the same one lies in the difficulty of the learning situation that results from these skill characteristics. When skill variations are controlled by different motor programs, this makes the learning situation more difficult. Thus, higher levels of contextual interference during practice are created by random practice, thereby establishing a more effortful processing situation than when skill variations are parameter modifications of the same motor program.

Changing motor programs from one trial to the next requires the restructuring of essential composite features of a skill, such as order of events, relative timing, and so on. On the other hand, modifying parameters of the same program is a relatively simple alteration that can be done with considerably less effort. Since an important feature of the contextual interference effect is that higher levels of contextual interference requires learners to engage in more effortful learning processes, it seems likely that the types of skill related changes demanded from trial to trial should influence the degree of contextual interference created by manipulating practice schedules.

Experience and Open Skills. Another situation that appears to influence the degree of the effect of contextual interference is experience. This factor seems to be particularly interactive when the skill being learned is an open skill. In the language of motor learning, an open skill is one in which the object of the action is moving and must be acted on according to the dictates of its time and space characteristics. Examples here include hitting a pitched ball in baseball, catching a thrown ball, and returning a serve in tennis. For open skills, it appears that prior experience with the space/time prediction feature of these skills is important for achieving the benefits of contextual interference.

An example of an experiment that illustrates this situation is one reported by Del Rey (1989). Subjects from a beginning tennis class were given specific training about predicting a moving object while subjects from a beginning jogging class were not given any information about such prediction. Then both groups were given practice performing a coincidence-anticipation timing task in which four different stimulus speeds were practiced following either a random or a blocked schedule.

Results of both retention and transfer tests showed the random practice benefit only for the trained subjects. What is notable about these results is that in prior experiments using an anticipation timing task, the contextual interference effect typically was not found (Del Rey, Wughalter, DuBois, & Carnes, 1982; Edwards, Elliott, & Lee, 1986). Thus the experience factor appears to be pertinent for learning variations of this type of skill.

It is possible, then, that learning skill variations demanded by open skills require a practice schedule organization scheme that differs from closed skills. This may be due to the unique perception/action linkage associated with open skills, in which constant adaptability to an ever-changing environment is required for successful performance. This characteristic demands that both perceptual and motor components of the skill must be varied to some extent when these skills are performed. Thus, as Magill and Hall (1990) have proposed, it seems plausible that open skills in particular require that before learners experience the type of variability provided by high contextual interference practice schedules, they need to "get the idea of the movement," as Gentile (1972) phrased the initial stage of learning.

The important condition here is that the learner develop the capability of relating relevant environmental cues to specific movement patterns. Thus, early in practice, the practice schedule should provide the opportunity for establishing basic movement patterns and learning relevant environmental cues. This goal may best be accomplished by scheduling early practice sessions that involve blocks of trials of each skill variation being learned. Later in practice, with its emphasis on adapting the established movement patterns to the ever-changing environment characteristic of open skills, a more random type of practice schedule would be preferred.

The results of the Del Rey (1989) experiment described earlier provide some degree of support for this possibility. Even stronger support has been provided recently from an experiment by Goode and Wei (1988), in which early blocked practice followed by later random practice was better than either all random or all blocked practice for learning an anticipation timing skill.

Theoretical Implications

As a learning phenomenon, the contextual interference effect suggests that practice under high levels of contextual interference engages a person in fundamentally different learning processes than under lower levels. Thus this effect has distinct implications for motor learning theory, as theoretical accounts must be developed to explain why learning is affected by these practice schedule manipulations. In the preceding sections of this discussion, the point was made that higher levels of contextual interference seem to benefit learning because they require the learner to engage in more effortful learning processes during practice.

Although these more effortful processes may retard performance during practice compared to less effortful processes, they benefit learning, as demonstrated by performance on later retention and transfer tests. The theoretical issue here, then, is the need to identify these learning processes. At present, two views have emerged as the primary proposals of the characteristics of these processes. These two views will now be addressed briefly.

Distinctive and Elaborative Processing. Following the lead provided by Battig in explaining the contextual interference effect, Shea and his colleagues (Shea & Morgan, 1979; Shea & Zimny, 1983, 1988) have argued that increasing contextual interference increases the amount of multiple and variable encoding of information that occurs during learning. The result is that a more distinctive and elaborative memory representation of the skills is developed during practice.

Multiple and variable encodings result from the learner engaging in more and different strategies during practice to learn the skill variations. This in turn develops a memorial representation in which each skill variation is more distinct and elaborate. Distinctiveness refers to the unique characteristics that set the representation of one skill apart from that of another. Elaboration refers to the number of attributes associated with the representation of the skill as well as the operations involved in developing that representation.

The argument is that since during random practice different skill variations are in working memory simultaneously, they can be compared and contrasted more effectively than in blocked practice wherein direct comparisons of the skill variations occur very infrequently during practice.

Evidence supporting this view has been strongest when one of two approaches has been taken. One approach has been to record subjects' reports of the strategies they use during practice to learn the different skill variations (e.g., Shea & Zimny, 1983, 1988). When subjects tell what they are doing, it is clear that those in a random practice schedule are engaged in a number of different learning strategies to aid their learning. Included in these are strategies in which deliberate attempts are made to compare and contrast the different skill variations being practiced. The amount and type of strategies engaged in by subjects in random practice schedules differ from those in blocked schedules.

The other approach for testing this view of the contextual interference effect has been to engage subjects in a blocked schedule in the strategies that are considered to be characteristic of subjects in a random schedule (e.g., Wright, 1988). The prediction here is that subjects will benefit from these strategies so that learning in blocked practice schedules will become similar to those in random schedules. In the experiment by Wright (1988), this procedure was successful in enabling the blocked schedule condition to achieve random schedule learning outcomes.

Action Plan Reconstruction View. An alternative to the distinctiveness/elaboration process activities view was offered by Lee and Magill (1983, 1985). They argued that high contextual interference practice schedules lead to an increase in effortful processing activity because, on a given practice trial, previously encoded information about the skill variation being practiced has been partially or completely forgotten. This forgetting is due to interference from having to perform the other skill variations on trials that intervened since the last trial of that particular skill variation. As a result of this forgetting, the learner must reconstruct partially or completely an action plan appropriate for performing that particular skill variation.

This differs from what occurs in low contextual interference practice situations. Since the same skill variation will be performed several times in succession, the same action plan can be kept active and only slight modifications are needed from trial to trial. While this latter situation is more effective for enhancing skill performance during practice, it leads to a poorly developed memory representation, which is evidenced by poor performance on later retention and transfer tests.

The stronger memory representation that leads to better retention is the result of the more effortful processing required by the action plan reconstruction that is required by high contextual interference practice schedules. Better novel transfer performance results from the similarity of processing demands during practice and transfer (Kolers & Roediger, 1984; Lee, 1988).

The notion of the action plan here is related to what a person must create just prior to initiating any action. First, there must be a retrieval of the appropriate generalized motor program related to the intended action. Since this program only contains certain invariant features of the action, specific movement parameters must be added to meet the demands of the conditions of the "right now" action situation. Thus, on any practice trial an action plan must be created. What appears to differ for high and low contextual interference situations is the degree of construction, or reconstruction, that must occur.

Evidence supporting the action plan reconstruction view has been provided by two approaches that relate the contextual interference practice situation to a well-established memory phenomenon known as the spacing-of-repetitions effect (Hintzman, 1974; Melton, 1967). One approach has been to use a variation of the traditional short-term memory paradigm (e.g., Lee & Weeks, 1987; Weeks, Lee, & Elliott, 1987).

In these experiments, the movement to be recalled is first presented; then one group may experience an attention-demanding activity during a long retention interval while another group engages in no activity during a short retention interval. Then a recall test is given to both groups. But rather than stop here, a second retention interval is used with interpolated activity for both groups. This is then followed by another recall test.

Results of this procedure show that more forgetting occurs on the first recall test for the group that engaged in the retention interval activity than for the other group. However, on the second recall test the group that engaged in activity during the first retention interval shows an improvement and performs better than the other group. Thus the interpolated activity negatively affected performance for the short term but was a benefit for later memory performance.

The second approach has been to use a learning paradigm in which the practice trials for a skill are interpolated with different amounts of time and activity (e.g., Meeuwsen, 1987). Conditions of massed practice become similar to blocked practice in this paradigm, while more distributed practice can be similar to random practice or can have interpolated activity designed to produce trial-to-trial forgetting.

Results of this approach have been mixed. Meeuwsen (1987) showed that for retention, no differences occurred for spaced and nonspaced practice, regardless of the characteristics of the activity interpolated between spaced trials. However, for novel transfer, performance was significantly better for spaced than for nonspaced practice conditions.

A comment about the two explanation alternatives: It is clear that neither view which is proposed to explain why the contextual interference effect occurs has unequivocal support. While there is some support for both views, much remains to be done before a well-developed theoretical accounting of the contextual interference effect is established. Theoretical accounts of learning processes involved in motor skill learning need to take into account the contextual interference phenomenon. However, at present much remains to be investigated before such an accounting can be provided.

Practical Implications

Since the contextual interference effect is directly related to the organization of practice schedules for learning skill variations, it is relatively easy to develop specific practical applications concerning this effect. The most obvious one involves the scheduling of practice for situations in which variations of a skill must be learned in a specific amount of time.

An example would be the limited amount of time available for practice prior to a scheduled competition. The goal of the coach and athlete in this situation is to learn these skills as well as possible in the practice time available. Based on results of research investigating contextual interference, certain practice schedules will enable the coach and athlete to achieve this goal better than others.

When new skills are being learned, specific guidelines can be established for organizing effective practice schedules. If the skill variations to be learned require the athlete to perform distinctively different movement patterns for each variation, such as for different serves in tennis or badminton, different pitches in baseball, or perhaps even different plays in basketball or football, then increased amounts of contextual interference in practice will enhance the learning of these skills, even with beginners.

It may not be practical to employ random practice routines similar to those used in experiments investigating the contextual interference effect. However, recall that contextual interference is a continuum ranging from low to high amounts of interference. Blocked practice for each skill variation exemplifies the low end of the interference continuum while a trial-by-trial based random practice schedule represents an extreme high interference end of the continuum.

Thus the coach is free to experiment with a number of variations of practice schedules that will increase the amount of contextual interference and yet be practical to employ. For example, one skill variation could be practiced for a specific amount of time, such as for 10 minutes, then another could be practiced, and so on, for a specified amount of time in each practice session. These 10-minute blocks could be randomly organized in each session.

Another guideline relates to learning new skill variations of an open skill, such as learning to hit different pitches in baseball or return different serves in tennis or badminton. The best practice schedule appears to be one in which practice is initially more blocked, and then, after the basic movement pattern is established and critical perceptual cues have been identified, more randomized practice schedules should be introduced.

Finally, the contextual interference effect also has implications for practice in which skills are well learned but the goal of practice is to enhance those skills in preparation for upcoming competitions. This view of contextual interference extends the traditional way in which it has been considered, which has been to focus on learning new skills. A recent research example indicates how contextual interference can be incorporated into a practice routine for this type of situation.

An experiment by Hall, Cavazos, and Domingues (1991) investigated different levels of contextual interference in extra batting practice for a top-level junior college baseball team. Players received two extra batting practice sessions of 45 pitches for 2 days each week for 6 weeks. Each session consisted of 15 fastballs, 15 curves, and 15 change-ups. Based on a pretest, three groups were formed. One group hit following a blocked schedule of 15 of one pitch per block. A second group hit following a random schedule of the three pitches. The third group was a control group that did not take the extra batting practice.

Results of a 45-pitch posttest, presented randomly to simulate game conditions, indicated that the random practice group had significantly more solid hits, the dependent measure used for this study. Also, pre- to posttest improvement showed that the random practice group improved 56.7% while the blocked practice group improved only 24.8%. The extra batting practice obviously helped, as the control group improved only 6.2%. Thus, practice schedule organization can be seen as an important component in the process of preparing athletes to perform well-learned skills in an upcoming competition.

Conclusion

While motor learning research has historically claimed that its results have implications for enhancing sport performance, few effects appear to have as clear an implication as the contextual interference effect. The significance of this effect is that it demonstrates there is more to increasing skill learning or enhancing preparation for an upcoming competition than the amount of practice engaged in.

The contextual interference effect provides an effective argument that the practice schedule is also a critical variable for achieving these learning and performance goals. What may be unnerving about this effect from an applied perspective is that its implications for designing practice sessions to enhance sport performance are counterintuitive. That is, better performance results when the amount of interference during practice is increased.

Whereas intuition might suggest that practicing several closely related skills in a random schedule would introduce interference that would hinder learning, the contextual interference effect provides evidence that in many cases this type of increased interference is beneficial. In fact, the more traditional low interference based practice organization schemes appear to produce more negative outcomes than beneficial ones.

References

Adams, J.A. (1987). Historical review and appraisal of research on the learning, retention, and transfer of human motor skills. *Psychological Bulletin*, **101**, 41-74.

Battig, W.F. (1966). Facilitation and interference. In E.A. Bilodeau (Ed.), Acquisition of *skill* (pp. 215-244). New York: Academic Press.

Battig, W.F. (1972). Intratask interference as a source of facilitation in transfer and retention. In R.F. Thompson & J.F. Voss (Eds.), *Topics in learning and performance* (pp. 131-159). New York: Academic Press.

Battig, W.F. (1979). The flexibility of human memory. In L.S. Cermak & F.I.M. Craik (Eds.), *Levels of processing in human memory* (pp. 23-44). Hillsdale, NJ: Erlbaum.

Del Rey, P. (1989). Training and contextual interference effects on memory and transfer. *Research Quarterly for Exercise and Sport*, **60**, 342-347.

Del Rey, P., Wughalter, E., DuBois, D., & Carnes, M. (1982). Effects of contextual interference and retention intervals on transfer. *Perceptual and Motor Skills*, **54**, 467-476.

Edwards, J.M., Elliott, D., & Lee, T.D. (1986). Contextual interference effects during skill acquisition and transfer in Down's syndrome adolescents. *Adapted Physical Activity Quarterly*, **3**, 250-258.

Gentile, A.M. (1972). A working model of skill acquisition with application to teaching. *Quest*, **17**, 3-23.

Gentner, D.R. (1987). Timing of skilled performance: Tests of the proportional duration model. *Psychological Review*, **94**, 225-276.

Gentner, D.R. (1988). Observed movements reflect both central and peripheral mechanisms: A reply to Heuer. *Psychological Review*, **95**, 558.

Goode, S.L., & Magill, R.A. (1986). Contextual interference effects in learning three badminton serves. *Research Quarterly for Exercise and Sport*, **57**, 308-314.

Goode, S.L. & Wei, P. (1988). Differential effect of variations of random and blocked practice on novices learning an open motor skill [Abstract]. In D.L. Gill & J.E. Clark (Eds.), *Abstracts of Research Papers, 1988* (p. 230). American Alliance for Health, Physical Education, Recreation and Dance annual convention, Kansas City. Reston, VA: AAHPERD.

Hall, K.G., Cavazos, R., & Domingues, D.A. (1991, June). *The effects of contextual interference on extra batting practice.* Paper presented at the annual conference of the North American Society for the Psychology of Sport and Physical Activity, Asilomar, CA.

Heuer, H. (1988). Testing the invariance of relative timing: Comment on Gentner. *Psychological Review*, **97**, 492-497.

Heuer, H., & Schmidt, R.A. (1988). Transfer of learning among motor patterns with different relative timing. *Journal of Experimental Psychology: Human Perception and Performance*, **14**, 249-252.

Hintzman, D.L. (1974). Theoretical implications of the spacing effect. In R.L. Solso (Ed.), *Theories in cognitive psychology: The Loyola Symposium* (pp. 77-99). Potomac, MD: Erlbaum.

Jelsma, O., & Pieters, J.M. (1989). Practice schedule and cognitive style interaction in learning a maze task. *Applied Cognitive Psychology*, **3**, 73-83.

Kolers, P.O., & Roediger, H.L. III (1984). Procedures of mind. *Journal of Verbal Learning and Verbal Behavior*, **23**, 425-449.

Lee, T.D. (1988). Transfer appropriate processing: A framework for conceptualizing practice effects in motor learning. In O.G. Meijer & K. Roth (Eds.), *Complex movement behaviour: 'The' motor-action controversy* (pp. 201-215). Amsterdam: North-Holland.

Lee, T.D., & Magill, R.A. (1983). The locus of contextual interference in motor-skill acquisition. *Journal of Experimental Psychology: Learning, Memory, and Cognition*, **9**, 730-746.

Lee, T.D., & Magill, R.A. (1985). Can forgetting facilitate skill acquisition? In D. Goodman, R.B. Wilberg, & I.M. Franks (Eds.), *Differing perspectives in motor learning, memory, and control* (pp. 3-22). Amsterdam: North-Holland.

Lee, T.D., & Weeks, D.J. (1987). The beneficial influence of forgetting on short-term retention of movement information. *Human Movement Science*, **6**, 233-245.

Magill, R.A. (1989). *Motor learning: Concepts and applications* (3rd ed.). Dubuque, IA: W.C. Brown.

Magill, R.A., & Hall, K.G. (1990). A review of the contextual interference effect in motor skill acquisition. *Human Movement Science*, **9**, 241-289.

Meeuwsen, H.J. (1987). *Spacing of repetitions and the contextual interference effect in motor skill learning.* Unpublished doctoral dissertation, Louisiana State University.

Melton, A.W. (1967). Repetition and retrieval from memory. *Science*, **158**, 532.

Pigott, R.E., & Shapiro, D.C. (1984). Motor schema: The structure of the variability session. *Research Quarterly for Exercise and Sport*, **55**, 41-45.

Poto, C.C. (1988). *How forgetting facilitates remembering: An analysis of the contextual interference effect in motor learning.* Unpublished doctoral dissertation, Louisiana State University.

Salmoni, A.W., Schmidt, R.A., & Walter, C.B. (1984). Knowledge of results and motor learning: A review and reappraisal. *Psychological Bulletin*, **95**, 355-386.

Schmidt, R.A. (1975). A schema theory of discrete motor skill learning. *Psychological Review*, **82**, 225-260.

Schmidt, R.A. (1988). *Motor control and learning* (2nd ed.). Champaign, IL: Human Kinetics.

Shea, J.B., & Morgan, R.L. (1979). Contextual interference effects on the acquisition, retention, and transfer of a motor skill. *Journal of Experimental Psychology: Human Learning and Memory*, **5**, 179-187.

Shea, J.B., & Zimny, S.T. (1983). Context effects in memory and learning movement information. In R.A. Magill (Ed.), *Memory and control of action* (pp. 345-366). Amsterdam: North-Holland.

Shea, J.B., & Zimny, S.T. (1988). Knowledge incorporation in motor representation. In O.G. Meijer & K. Roth (Eds.), *Complex movement behaviour: 'The' motor-action controversy* (pp. 289-314). Amsterdam: North-Holland.

Tolman, E.C. (1932). *Purposive behavior in animals and man.* New York: Century.

Weeks, D.J., Lee, T.D., & Elliott, D. (1987). Differential forgetting and spacing effects in short-term motor memory. *Journal of Human Movement Studies*, **13**, 309-321.

Whitehurst, M., & Del Rey, P. (1983). Effects of contextual interference, task difficulty, and levels of processing on pursuit tracking. *Perceptual and Motor Skills*, **57**, 619-628.

Wood, C.A., & Ging, C.A. (1991). The role of interference and task similarity on the acquisition, retention, and transfer of simple motor skills. *Research Quarterly for Exercise and Sport*, **62**, 18-26.

Wright, D. (1988). *Acquisition and retention of a motor skill as a function of intra-task and inter-task processing.* Unpublished doctoral dissertation, The Pennsylvania State University.

Practice: A Search for Task Solutions

Karl M. Newell and Paul V. McDonald
University of Illinois at Urbana–Champaign

Practice makes perfect is an adage advanced in many walks of life. In reality, however, even if we could define perfection as an attainable state in motor skill acquisition, practice is to be understood as a necessary but not sufficient condition for its realization. It is the structure of practice and how it relates to the organismic, environmental, and task constraints that determines in part the attainment of a potential solution to a task goal.

Magill has emphasized one instance of the many variables that can influence the structure of practice and the resultant motor learning and performance. The focus is contextual interference (Magill & Hall, 1990), a kind of intertask facilitation effect, introduced to the motor learning domain by Shea and Morgan (1979). There are many other practice variables that influence motor learning, however, including the amount of practice (e.g., number of trials), the practice and rest relations (e.g., massed vs. distributed practice), the nature of the augmented information available (e.g., demonstrations, feedback), and the relation of practice tasks to other activities of daily living (e.g., other tasks within or between the practice sessions).

All of the foregoing variables, which are by no means inclusive, combine to shape and alter the structure of practice and the acquisition of skill. These practice variables are the kinds of factors that instructors in a variety of physical activity subdomains such as dance, sport, or work need to understand in order to structure practice in a principled way to facilitate motor skill acquisition and performance.

In this commentary on Magill's review of the role of contextual interference for enhancing motor skill learning and performance, we are going to reexamine the nature and scope of the contextual interference effect. We will then elaborate on some empirical and theoretical reservations with respect to the generalizability of the contextual interference effect. Finally, we will briefly introduce some theorizing as to ways in which we might usefully consider the process of practice, a perspective that will also offer a different approach to considering the contextual interference phenomenon.

It is a surprising and somewhat telling comment that our understanding of practice effects in motor learning and performance is less than adequate. There is still a tendency to accept the general notion of more being better, with very little research directed to understanding the influence of the structure and quality of practice per se on motor skill acquisition. Of course it takes considerable time and energy to conduct investigations of practice effects, particularly if they are viewed in the long term. The operational demands of realistic practice studies have contributed to the rather short-term nature of so-called motor learning studies over the last several decades. However, there appears currently to be an increased sensitivity to the problems associated with a short-term approach to the study of motor learning. The work of Shea and Magill on contextual interference contributes to refocusing our efforts on the general problem of practice as a very important variable for motor skill acquisition.

The Contextual Interference Effect

The contextual interference phenomenon is basically one in which the practice structure of different tasks influences the acquisition of, or performance on, those tasks. In particular, if one wishes to learn Tasks A, B, and C, then the contextual interference effect suggests that practicing these tasks in some random (non-blocked) as opposed to sequential (blocked) fashion facilitates the acquisition of each task, even on a retention test. There also appear to be some transfer advantages from following a random acquisition schedule of Tasks A, B, and C when attempting a task criterion that was not part of the task sequence practiced earlier. An additional implication is that even if one wishes to learn only Task A, there might be some benefits to learning Tasks B and C at the same time with a random practice schedule.

The advantages of contextual interference in acquisition have been demonstrated in a number of studies, and Magill and Hall (1990) have recently reviewed these findings in detail. The effect seems to be real, holds a certain degree of generalizability across tasks, and is an interesting phenomenon that needs to be accounted for in our understanding of motor skill acquisition. Magill also suggests in his target article for this commentary that contextual interference might be used as a potential strategy for enhancing performance in sport skills.

The Generalizability of Contextual Interference

Although the contextual interference effect seems to hold some degree of generalizability, there are various limitations to this effect on a number of different dimensions. Magill mentioned some of these in his talk, but we would like to highlight a number of empirical and theoretical problems. We begin with the empirical reservations.

Empirical Reservations

One limitation that Magill identified and that appears to be particularly problematic is the degree to which the effect is task limited or task specific. That is, contextual interference may well be limited to transfer effects between certain kinds of task constraints. Magill organizes these task-limited findings under the *movement class* concept of Schmidt's (1975) schema theory. Unfortunately, movement class was never adequately defined in the schema theory, and consequently this particular approach to task classification inevitably holds a number of problems. The claim is that contextual interference facilitates *between* movement class transfer, whereas it appears to have weaker or no effects in a *within* movement class transfer situation.

Clearly, a major factor in any attempt to identify task generalizability is the scheme used to categorize tasks. Fleischman and Quaintance (1984) have synthesized the many approaches to task analysis. Most classification schemes are no more than descriptions of tasks on some (often poorly) defined dimension of the behavior. The within and between movement class distinction used by Magill falls into this category. The general problem is that the functional role of task constraints in motor control has been sought from the a priori descriptive categories of motor tasks rather than the task descriptions being formulated a posteriori on the basis of an understanding of the role that task constraints play in motor control (Newell, 1989).

The contextual interference phenomenon also appears to be limited to the adult segment of the population in that the few studies which have examined this effect in children have found weaker or nonexistent effects. This is interesting because it is counter to the schema theory based proposal that the variability of practice effects are much stronger in children than in adults (Shapiro & Schmidt, 1982).

On the other hand, this age related difference is consistent with the general notion of a between- versus a within-class consideration of the contextual interference effect. This is because schema theory advanced projections about variability and transfer on a within-task basis whereas the contextual interference effect is advancing projections on a between-task basis. In short, there appears to be some age related mediation of the contextual interference effects that are presumably reflections of experiential or practice considerations, but these have yet to be developed much beyond intuition.

A final empirical limitation that we would like to highlight, and which is not mentioned in Magill's commentary, is whether the contextual interference effect is limited to a particular stage of practice. It should be recognized that all the studies demonstrating the contextual interference effect are limited to some middle stage of practice in a particular task setting.

A characterization of this stage is difficult to define, in part because stage concepts of skill acquisition are also poorly defined. However, Magill would surely not claim that the performers in the contextual interference studies to date are highly skilled at the particular task at hand, or that they are complete novices in the sense of being unable to produce some reasonably stable solution to the task demands at hand. The question remains, therefore, whether the contextual interference effect has some lasting influence through the early and more advanced stages of practice and, in general, all the various locations on the dynamic of learning a given task.

The above concern about the potential practice limitations of contextual interference is an empirical question. However, it would seem doubtful that the benefits derived from the contextual interference structure of practice would in fact be continued throughout a lengthy practice schedule. Athletes in particular perform thousands, and perhaps millions, of trials on a particular skill during their respective careers. The contextual interference manipulation as studied to date has only tapped into a particular stage of the practice phenomenon. Thus it seems premature for Magill to suggest that contextual interference manipulations might be used as a potential strategy for enhancing performance in sport.

These limitations in our understanding of task, individual differences, and practice effects all present some boundary conditions to the generalizability of the contextual interference effect. The degree to which these are meaningful comes down in part to understanding the impact of task, subject experience, and practice. These issues are significant problems for the motor skill acquisition domain in general. To suggest that transfer effects are only as good as our understanding of tasks is based on the premise that a broad theoretical perspective of task constraints will provide the foundation for generalizing the impact of tasks. This leads us to some theoretical reservations about contextual interference.

Theoretical Reservations

Magill has elaborated upon two potential hypotheses that have been put forward as a theoretical base for the contextual interference effect: the elaboration benefit explanation and the action plan reconstruction view (see Magill & Hall, 1990). We have a number of reservations which collectively suggest that further theoretical and empirical analysis may render these particular hypotheses as superfluous. That is, if we begin to examine the transfer effects of contextual interference from another point of view, then in fact the two hypotheses advanced may not be particularly useful and probably would not need to be postulated in the first place.

It is instructive to note that the studies which have examined the contextual interference effect all rest on the analysis of outcome scores. This of course is the standard, traditional behavioral experimental psychology approach to skill acquisition. The last 10 to 20 years, however, have demonstrated the relevance and importance of understanding the movement dynamics in relation to the skill acquisition problem.

The contextual interference phenomenon, like most phenomena in the skill acquisition domain, would be enhanced by an examination of the accompanying movement dynamics. For example, there may well be some significant changes in the movement dynamics that arise from the different practice structures (random vs. blocked), and they might render, for example, the so-called cognitive hypotheses of elaboration and reconstruction as superfluous.

An important theoretical problem, and one that is not limited to the contextual task interference effect but is of general significance for motor skill acquisition, is that in spite of the concern for the problem of task structure to skill acquisition, there is no development toward what might be called a theory of tasks. We have little understanding at this point as to how task constraints influence skill acquisition (Newell, 1989; Newell, van Emmerik, & McDonald, 1989). For example, in discussing how Task A might influence Task B, we have little more than a descriptive approach of tasks, often on some relatively poorly defined or undefined dimension.

Task constraints are only part of the confluence of constraints to action. The traditional approaches to defining task constraints that emphasize the observer oriented extrinsic constraints to a task may be a convenient initial step in task analysis (Fleischman & Quaintance, 1984), but not sufficient for describing and understanding the influence of task constraints on motor skill acquisition.

The approach within our developing framework for motor skill acquisition is to have the task constraints, in addition to organismic and environmental constraints, constructing a perceptual-motor workspace in which the dynamics arising in this workspace are emergent properties from the confluence of constraints imposed (Newell, Kugler, P.N., van Emmerik, R.E.A., & McDonald, P.V., 1989; Newell, McDonald, & Kugler, 1991). This approach suggests that even a full analysis of the extrinsic task dimensions will not be sufficient for understanding the performer's perception of the dynamical similarity and dissimilarity that arises from the organism/environment interaction from different task structures. It will be the performer's perspective of these constraints, not the experimenter's extrinsic perspective of them, that needs to be understood in order to approach a general explanation of transfer effects.

A final and major theoretical reservation about the Magill commentary— and again this is not peculiar to the contextual interference effect—is that there is no real theory of practice in motor skill acquisition. That is, practice more often than not is discussed in a behavioral outcome orientation with little or no attention directed to what we call the *process* of practice. Thus, while practice influences performance scores over trials, and learning is an inference that is drawn from *changes* in performance over trials, there is surprisingly no theory of the process of practice. Theories of motor learning have tended to relate to the product rather than the process of practice.

The Process of Practice and the Nature of Task Constraints

Our understanding of the effect of practice per se on skill acquisition, and in particular how the structure of practice facilitates learning, could be approached by considering two important and related questions: What is the process of practice? What is the nature of tasks? These two thorny questions have plagued progress in understanding the role of practice effects per se in skill acquisition, in part because theoretical perspectives have not approached these questions head on. There are no direct answers at this time, but it would be useful to consider the questions from the following perspective.

Practice can be considered as a form of exploratory behavior, a continually evolving search for task solutions (Fowler & Turvey, 1978; Newell et al., 1989). Bernstein (1967, p. 134) captured an element of this perspective when he said,

> Practice . . . does not consist in repeating the means of solution of a motor problem time after time, but in the process of solving this problem again and again by techniques which we changed and perfected from repetition to repetition.

Thus, even though there may be repetition in terms of achieving a given task goal, there is not repetition to the solution of the motor problem. As Bernstein (1967, p. 134) went on to say, "practice is a particular type of repetition without repetition."

Practice may be viewed as the ongoing search for solutions in a perceptual-motor workspace that continuously evolves from the confluence of constraints arising from the learner, environment, and task (Fowler & Turvey, 1978; Newell et al., 1989). The schematic of Figure 1 shows the relation of the constraints to action and their influence on shaping the perceptual-motor workspace from which a given coordination mode arises. In this approach, practice involves the

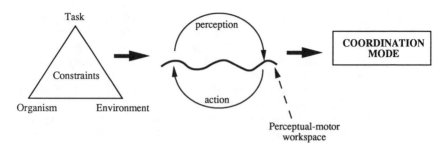

Figure 1 — A schematic of the relation of constraints to action, the perceptual-motor workspace, and the emergent coordination mode.

exploration and exploitation of the evolving dynamics in the perceptual-motor workspace. One of the keys to skilled performance is learning to take advantage of the natural dynamics that exist in the perceptual-motor workspace.

The constraints to action may be categorized on the basis of whether they arise from the organism, the environment, or the task (Newell, 1986). The many sources of constraint in each category interact to provide a confluence of constraints to the evolving movement sequence that is produced within a specific task context. In this view, constraints act to channel rather than specify the movement dynamics. A key feature to this approach is to formally identify the nature and influence of the various sources of constraint to action. The influence of task properties as a potentially organizing source of constraint to motor skill acquisition has not been afforded the emphasis it should in extant accounts of motor learning and control (Newell, 1989).

It is useful to consider the perceptual-motor workspace as an interface between the kinematics of information and the kinetics of action. Consequently, learning is synonymous with an increase in the coordination of the mapping of the kinematic informational properties with the kinetic motor properties in realization of the task demands (Shaw & Alley, 1985). A key feature of this approach, then, is understanding the cyclic nature of how information in the perceptual flows contributes to channeling the search through the dynamics that arise from attempts to satisfy the goal demands, together with the form of information generated by actions aimed at realizing the goal demands.

This interface of the perceptual-motor workspace is dynamic, that is, its structure is time varying and its surface is a changing multidimensional structure of equilibrium regions and gradients. Different tasks harness or focus on different portions of the perceptual-motor workspace and ultimately provide different boundaries to the regions of that workspace which need to be explored and exploited to satisfy the task demands.

The approach to understanding tasks may be sought at different levels of analysis. To reiterate, an important and perhaps first step might be to more formally classify tasks on their extrinsic dimensions. Task description and analysis has proved to be a continual challenge in motor skills, and most task categories are ambiguous or, at best, descriptive (Fleischman & Quaintance, 1984). A key to analyzing tasks is to describe them in the dimensions that map directly into the dynamics of action (McGinnis & Newell, 1982; Saltzman & Kelso, 1987).

Given that task constraints interact with those arising from the organism and environment to determine the dynamic interface of the perceptual-motor workspace, a second step in pursuing a theory of tasks is to understand how the extrinsic dimensions of tasks serve to channel the dynamics of the perceptual-motor workspace as perceived by the performer. The concept of the perceptual-motor workspace may ultimately prove more useful in understanding task structure than the extrinsic dimensions that are more obvious to an observer, such as an experimenter. This approach to task structure is an enormous challenge but one that appears promising, particularly as it dovetails with a dynamic approach to considering both the coordination and control of movement and the process of motor skill acquisition.

The dynamical landscape at the perception/action interface can be approached through considering probabilistic states of attractor dynamics as building-blocks for the organization of action and the search for solutions to the task constraints (Newell et al., 1989; Schöner, 1989). These attractor states of the perceptual-motor workspace help to provide formal principled solutions for accommodating several traditional problems in motor learning and control. These principles include a reduction of the degrees of freedom requiring control in contrast to those apparent at the behavioral level, and a mechanism for accommodating the dynamical features that are evident in movement control. The search through the perceptual-motor workspace may be categorized as an exploration for a more appropriate mapping of the perceptual information flows and the action energetic flows.

In short, the learner has what the artificial inelligence community has called a high-dimensional optimization problem, although whether optimal or merely robust solutions are sought in biological search strategies remains an open issue. How the subject searches through the paths of the various control spaces is the centerpiece of the problem of search strategies and the heart of the process of practice (Newell et al., 1989). Search strategies in learning have been largely ignored through the predominant focus on the relative size of the change in the movement outcome scores and the indifference to considering trial-to-trial or within-trial relations of performance.

Thus, in summary, we suggest that task structure in practice channels the search for task solutions in mapping perception and action. There are several important elements in developing this orientation to motor skill acquisition that include understanding (a) the nature of the perceptual-motor workspace, (b) the way in which information arises from the workspace, (c) how augmented information may channel the search, (d) and finally, the generic features of search strategies used by subjects in searching for solutions to task goals. We anticipate that this approach to motor skill acquisition will directly open up the process of practice and the role that task constraints play in structuring practice (Newell et al., 1989, 1991).

Contextual Interference in Context

The above is only a brief outline of our approach to practice as an ongoing search strategy, but it provides a sufficient basis for reconsidering various issues that relate to the structure of practice. Furthermore, we can formulate a framework for how task structures interact to determine the learning and performance of motor skills. In particular, given the focus of this commentary, one might reexamine the role of the contextual interference effect in light of the theoretical framework briefly sketched.

One limitation of the motor skill acquisition area is our shallow understanding of task structure, and this is particularly evident in the contextual interference literature. That is, there is no formal basis for determining what is within or between a movement class structure. A dynamical approach to motor skill acquisition suggests that an understanding of transfer, positive or negative, is more usefully sought at the level of the emergent dynamics in the perceptual-motor workspace rather than an analysis of the extrinsic task dimensions. To the extent that transfer can be predicted from traditional extrinsic task dimensions, it is because of a correlation between these dimensions and the attractor layout (in terms of equilibrium regions and gradients) of the perceptual-motor workspace.

Imposing modified task constraints in a practice schedule requires the performer to search through different or additional properties of the perceptual-motor workspace. This task-imposed channeling of the search behavior may afford additional information for the performer to more fully perceive the layout of the perceptual-motor workspace. Thus, performance facilitation could arise from multiple task criteria in practice because the learner has developed a fuller understanding of the dynamics of the perceptual-motor workspace. This more complete characterization of the workspace leads to a more efficient and effective search through the space for task-appropriate solutions.

Thus one does not need to invoke either of the hypotheses summarized by Magill (Magill, this volume; Magill & Hall, 1990) to account for the empirical effect called contextual interference. This is because the modified task structures in blocked and random variations of task constraints lead to different information about the perceptual-motor workspace being available to the learners. This differential information about the perceptual-motor workspace from the task structures affords the basis for different output in terms of action.

The elaboration-benefits explanation and the action plan reconstruction view represent proposed information processing activity farther down the information processing line (in terms of input through output) than information input. Thus, these cognitive processing views of contextual interference may be superfluous in light of the different information that is available to be picked up from the different perceptual-motor workspace dynamics, prior to cognitive transformations.

The act of searching the workspace itself also changes the layout of the workspace. This feature contributes to the nonstationarity of the workspace and its continually evolving dynamic surface. Thus, searching for task solutions through practice is a process that may realize a current task solution but one that also influences the nature of subsequent searches through the workspace. This principle holds direct relevance to the traditional problems of transfer (positive and negative) and interference (proactive or retroactive) in motor skill learning.

Task structure in a practice session acts as a constraint that channels the search through the perceptual-motor workspace. The organization of task structures through a session or over sessions of directed practicing is no more than a larger scale notion over a broader time span of this basic proposal. We anticipate that approaching practice as a search through the perceptual-motor workspace for task solutions will not only lead us to new ways to consider motor learning but also the transfer and retention effects, such as realized through the task structures of what have been labeled contextual interference.

References

Bernstein, N.A. (1967). *The co-ordination and regulation of movements*. London: Pergamon.

Fleischman, E.A., & Quaintance, M.K. (1984). *Taxonomies of human performance*. New York: Academic Press.

Fowler, C.A., & Turvey, M.T. (1978). Skill acquisition: An event approach with special reference to searching for the optimum of a function of several variables. In G.E. Stelmach (Ed.), *Information processing in motor control and learning* (pp. 1-40). New York: Academic Press.

Magill, R.A., & Hall, K.G. (1990). A review of the contextual interference effect in motor skill acquisition. *Human Movement Science*, **9**, 241-289.

McGinnis, P.M., & Newell, K.M. (1982). Topological dynamics: A framework for describing movement and its constraints. *Human Movement Science*, **1**, 289-305.

Newell, K.M. (1986). Constraints on the development of coordination. In M.G. Wade & H.T.A. Whiting (Eds.), *Motor development in children: Aspects of coordination and control* (pp. 341-360). Boston: Martinus Nijhoff.

Newell, K.M. (1989). On task and theory specificity. *Journal of Motor Behavior*, **21**, 92-96.

Newell, K.M., Kugler, P.N., van Emmerik, R.E.A., & McDonald, P.V. (1989). Search strategies and the acquisition of coordination. In S.A. Wallace (Ed.), *Perspectives on the coordination of movement* (pp. 85-122). Amsterdam: North-Holland.

Newell, K.M., van Emmerik, R.E.A., & McDonald, P.V. (1989). On simple movements and complex theories (and vice versa). *Behavioral and Brain Sciences*, **12**, 229-230.

Newell, K.M., McDonald, P.V., & Kugler, P.N. (1991). The perceptual-motor workspace and the acquisition of skill. In J. Requin & G.E. Stelmach (Eds.), *Tutorials in motor neuroscience* (pp. 95-108). Dordrecht: Kluwer.

Saltzman, E., & Kelso, J.A.S. (1987). Skilled actions: A task dynamic approach. *Psychological Review*, **94**, 84-106.

Schmidt, R.A. (1975). A schema theory of discrete motor skill learning. *Psychological Review*, **82**, 225-260.

Schöner, G. (1989). Learning and recall in a dynamic theory of coordination patterns. *Biological Cybernetics*, **62**, 39-54.

Shapiro, D.C., & Schmidt, R.A. (1982). The schema theory: Recent evidence and developmental implications. In J.A.S. Kelso & J.E. Clark (Eds.), *The development of movement control and co-ordination* (pp. 113-150). New York: Wiley.

Shaw, R.E., & Alley, T.R. (1985). How to draw learning curves: Their use and justification. In T.D. Johnson & A.T. Pietrewicz (Eds.), *Issues in the ecological study of learning* (pp. 275-304). Hillsdale: Erlbaum.

Shea, J.B., & Morgan, R.L. (1979). Contextual interference effects on the acquisition, retention, and transfer of a motor skill. *Journal of Experimental Psychology: Human Learning and Memory*, **5**, 179-187.

The Development of Gender Differences in Throwing: Is Human Evolution a Factor?

Jerry R. Thomas and Mary W. Marzke
Arizona State University

Gender differences, generally favoring boys, in motor performance (Thomas & French, 1985), physical performance (Smoll & Schutz, 1990), motor activity (Eaton & Enns, 1986), and physical activity (Thomas & Thomas, 1988) have been consistently reported across childhood and adolescence. Thomas and French (1985) identified the difference in boys' and girls' throwing for distance as being larger and earlier in development than any other motor performance skill. Subsequently, Nelson, Thomas, Nelson, and Abraham (1986) reported that a significant amount of the gender difference in throwing was accounted for by anthropometric characteristics they identified as biological.

In a 3-year longitudinal follow-up (Nelson, Thomas, & Nelson, 1991), they found that the differences between girls and boys became greater, mostly due to increasingly better throwing patterns for boys. The traditional view of form differences in throwing has been that girls lagged behind boys in development but the form of the movement was the same (Roberton, 1982). However, there is little evidence to substantiate this proposition. In fact, Rippee et al. (1991) suggested that girls did not lag behind boys but instead develop a poor throwing pattern and learn to use it more efficiently over practice. Actually, there is no published evidence that the throwing kinematics, ground reaction forces, or muscle EMG of expert males and females are similar or different.

Most explanations of gender differences prior to puberty in motor performance (Thomas & French, 1985), physical performance (Smoll & Schutz, 1990), physical activity (Thomas & Thomas, 1988), and motor activity (Eaton & Enns, 1986) have relied on different environmental treatments such as cultural norms, encouragement and practice, and treatment by parents, peers, teachers, and coaches. Postpuberty explanations have indicated an interaction between biological (due to growth hormones) and environmental factors as influencing performance (Smoll & Schutz, 1990; Thomas & French, 1985), particularly on tasks in which size, strength, and power are important.

However, Thomas and French (1985) suggested that biological factors might play an important role in the development of gender differences in overhand throwing, even prior to puberty. They came to this conclusion for several reasons: (a) effect sizes between boys and girls were three times larger than for other motor performance tasks; (b) cross-cultural studies report larger gender differences in throwing performance than for other tasks; (c) throwing is one of the most stable tasks (relative order of performers) across childhood; and (d) training studies do not reduce the gender differences in throwing as in most other motor performance tasks.

Based on such data, we believe that the literature on throwing as a factor in human evolution (e.g., Calvin, 1982, 1983a; Darlington, 1975; Isaac, 1987) has considerable implications for the current findings about the development of gender differences in throwing. Calvin (1982, 1983a) and Darlington (1975) have indicated that overhand throwing is a prime candidate for explaining rapid increases in brain size, redundancy, and lateralization in human evolution.

Throwing has a substantial growth curve based on the idea that "faster is bigger is better" (Calvin, 1982, 1983a); that is, throwing faster and farther has considerable advantage but requires increased neural brain circuitry to control the action. This is because overhand throwing requires rapid motor sequencing for a problem with three constraints: location of the person throwing (moving or stationary), location of the target (moving or stationary), and trajectory/velocity of the object being thrown.

Even if throwing is an important factor in human evolution, what is there about this record that suggests males should develop more skill in throwing than females? Were males more likely to be involved in aggressive encounters resulting in greater reproductive success for those who threw effectively? If women provided more child care, did carrying a young child rather than leaving her/him unattended influence the throwing motion (e.g., minimal differentiated trunk rotation)?

After a substantial review of the anthropological and historical records on throwing, Isaac (1987) concluded, "It will have been noted by the reader that all historical instances so far quoted relate to throwing by males, with the honourable exception of the Australian Aborigines. The implications of this will not be pursued here, but they are not unimportant" (p. 15).

In the following sections of this paper, we propose to (a) describe the gender differences in throwing as well as characteristics that relate to these differences such as puberty, kinematics, stability, training, and cross-cultural findings; (b) review the evidence from antiquity on gender differences in throwing, specifically the potential role of throwing in human evolution, evidence that early humans threw, contacts during exploration between Europeans and primative humans who threw, and possible explanations for the evolution of gender differences in throwing; (c) propose new approaches to this question that may yield additional information to confirm or refute the connections we have drawn between human evolution and the development of gender differences in throwing; and (d) suggest applications of these findings to developmental aspects of sport performance.

Gender Differences in Throwing

Considering the motor behavior of overhand throwing involves at least three levels of analysis: the outcome from the throw, for example the distance the ball traveled, ball velocity, or accuracy of the throw; the kinematics of the throwing movement qualitatively or quantitatively; and the control and coordination of the muscles involved in the throw, such as EMG activity in various muscle groups.

In addition, body characteristics associated with growth may influence the throwing movement, for example gender differences in height and weight, limb length, shoulder/hip ratio, and percent lean body mass. And of course environmental characteristics influence throwing, for example practice opportunities, encouragement, parental attitudes, instruction, and expectations. This section is organized around these general topics.

Performance Outcome in Throwing

Performance differences in overhand throwing between girls and boys across childhood and adolescence have been reported in numerous studies and summarized in many motor development textbooks. However, the most comprehensive summary is reported by Thomas and French (1985) in their meta-analysis of gender differences in motor performance.

Figure 1 depicts the standardized difference (called effect size) between boys and girls in throwing for distance. The solid line is the actual difference between girls and boys in standard deviation units where "0" represents no difference, positive values represent greater distances thrown by the boys, and negative

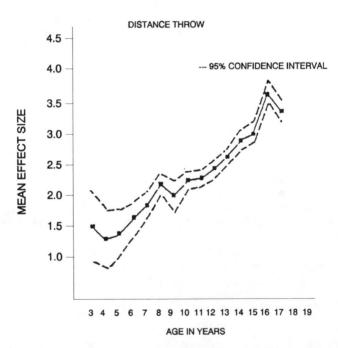

Figure 1 — Gender differences in throwing distance. Solid line represents difference (effect size) between males and females. Dotted lines are confidence intervals. From Thomas and French (1985, p. 268). Copyright 1985 by American Psychological Association. Reprinted with permission.

values represent greater distances thrown by the girls. The larger the standardized differences, the less overlap between the male and female distributions.

Note that in Figure 1, beginning at about 3 to 5 years of age, boys throw farther than girls by about 1.5 standard deviation units. That can be interpreted as the mean for boys' performance being shifted 1.5 standard deviations to the right of the mean for girls' performance, if you visualize a normal curve. Thus the left tail in the boys' distribution overlaps the right tail in the girls' distribution. The broken lines in Figure 1 are the confidence intervals for each point; the tighter they bound the curve, the more likely the curve provides an accurate estimate of performance.

By 16 to 18 years of age, the standardized difference in boys' and girls' throwing performance is about 3.5 standard deviation units, which can be interpreted as very little overlap between the two distributions. The data in Figure 1 are compiled from 11 studies producing 58 effect sizes based on 7,754 measurements for boys and 7,558 measurements for girls. (All measurements do not represent different boys and girls, as some are from cross-sectional studies of several age levels while others are from longitudinal studies that follow the same children across age.)

The gender differences in throwing performance at 3 to 5 years of age are three times (1.5 *SD* units vs. 0.5 *SD* units) the size of gender differences reported by Thomas and French (1985) for most other motor performance tasks (e.g., running speed, sit-ups, shuttle run, long jump, catching). Hardin and Garcia (1982) provide additional support for this. They report that from 6 to 9 years of age, girls' performance is 96 to 97% that of boys in the 50-yard dash, 90 to 95% in the standing long jump, but only 54 to 57% in the softball throw.

Gender differences in throwing performance are not unexpected; however, the size of the difference so early in life is exceptional, especially considering the smaller differences noted in other motor performance tasks. Why are these differences so great in throwing performance?

Throwing Form

Certainly, one explanation of the performance differences is that girls may use poorer throwing mechanics than boys. Data from form ratings at various ages tend to support this. For example, Roberton (1984), in the summaries of her work on throwing, provides developmental sequences for the throwing components of preparatory arm backswing, humerus action, forearm action, truck action, and foot action during various skill levels of the throwing movement. She notes that girls tend to lag behind boys in developing the various levels of each component. This idea is supported by Seefeldt and Haubenstricker (1982) in a total movement analysis of throwing in which they suggest that 60% of the boys in their study had developed mature throwing form by 5-1/2 years of age; 60% of the girls developed mature form by 8-1/2 years of age.

The basic assumption underlying both Roberton's and Seefeldt's work is that girls are developing through the same patterns for overhand throwing toward the same standard of throwing form. Is that a questionable assumption? Certainly girls and boys are both throwing overhand and the task has a similar objective: throwing with speed and accuracy. But is the mature pattern exhibited by the expert male and female the same?

Recently that assumption was questioned from two perspectives. Rippee et al. (1991) suggested "that many, if not most girls, simply get pretty good at throwing improperly . . . they can throw farther, faster and more accurately as they grow older, but only within the limits of their incorrect technique" (p. 184). Thomas, Thomas, and Gallagher (in press) have questioned whether the movement pattern of female and male experts is even the same.

For example, Figure 2 is from our work (Thomas, Thomas, Henrichs, Martin, & Marzke).[1] The data depicted are based on digitizing a 9-point total body model using data from three high-speed video cameras: Panel A is an All American male baseball player from Arizona State University, Panel B is an All American female softball player from Arizona State, Panel C is a 5-year-old boy, and Panel D is a 5-year-old girl. Several things might be noted from this qualita-

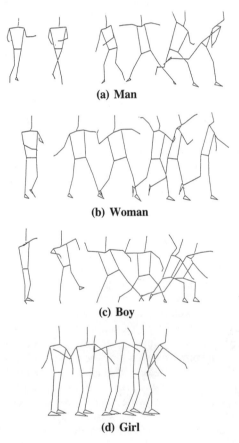

(a) Man

(b) Woman

(c) Boy

(d) Girl

Figure 2 — Stick figures of throwing.

---

[1]J.R. Thomas, K.T. Thomas, R. Henrichs, P. Martin, & M. Marzke. Research in progress, Arizona State University, Tempe.

tive analysis shown in Figure 2. First, the patterns of the female and male experts are not very similar. Second, the pattern of the 5-year-old boy looks more like that of the expert male than the pattern of the expert female does. Third, the 5-year-old girl's pattern is very different from the others.

Figure 2 is based on quantitative data (e.g., the 9-point body model that was digitized); however, our discussion about it was qualitative (e.g., the patterns look different). If we continue with a quantitative analysis of the female and male experts, there are at least two aspects of the pattern in which the kinematics of the movement differ.

Figure 3 represents the angle of twist for the male and female experts. Angle of twist is the difference in degrees between the shoulders and hips plotted against time. On the y-axis, "0" is shoulders and hips aligned, + angles means the shoulders are lagging behind the hips, and − angles means the shoulders are leading the hips. On the x-axis the black arrow at "0.0" is the point of ball release. The female expert has a lesser maximum angle of twist than the male, located at about 300 msec prior to ball release. This is basically where the arm and shoulder lag behind the hips as the hips begin their forward and counterclockwise rotation.

In the male expert, the maximum angle of twist is about 175 msec prior to ball release and the downward slope of the curve (angular velocity) is substan-

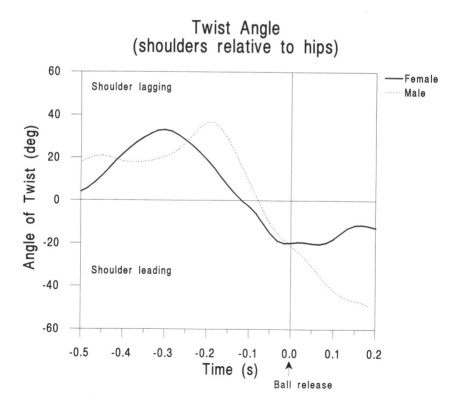

Figure 3 — Twist angle (shoulder relative to hips).

tially greater. This represents not only a greater amount of differentiation of the shoulders and hips but also a later and more rapid overtaking of the hips by the shoulders, producing more ball velocity. In addition, the male's shoulders continue to move in advance of the hips at follow-through.

The rate of rotation of the humerus about its long axis at the shoulder is called internal/external angular velocity. Figure 4 is the internal/external angular velocity of the humerus plotted against time. Notice that at 100 msec prior to ball release the male expert has a negative angular velocity of about 1,000 deg/sec where the female's angular velocity is about 0. The movement of the ball relative to the shoulder is such that the ball (and arm) lags more in the male. This is produced by external rotation of the humerus. However, note the male's very rapid increase to an internal rotation of 2,000 deg/sec at ball release where the female's increase in internal rotation is only to 1,000 deg/sec at ball release.

Thus the male has a much greater external-to-internal rotational rate, which produces about twice the angular velocity of the female at ball release. This can be conceived as a whip-like action in the arm as it overtakes the trunk at ball release to produce the high ball velocities observed in experts. However, this action appears to be considerably different in male and female experts.

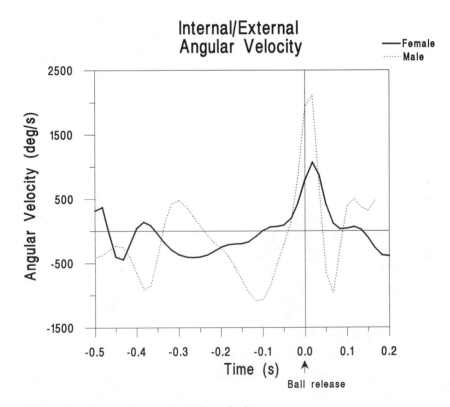

Figure 4 — Internal/external angular velocity.

Of course this is a small amount of quantitative data, but it is based on a number of trials of very expert overhand throwers. The data suggest to us that indeed the throwing patterns of male and female experts may be different. However, a final judgment will have to await our analysis of the additional data that we are currently completing on the experts and children.

Characteristics That Influence Throwing Performance

Biology. Thomas and French (1985) suggested that throwing was the only task from their meta-analysis in which biology might play a major role in gender differences prior to puberty (but for another view, see Smoll & Schutz, 1990). In following up this idea, Nelson et al. (1986) collected throwing performance and anthropometric data on 100 kindergartners (48 girls and 52 boys). Girls ($M = 4.8$ m, $SD = 1.4$ m) threw only 57% of the distance thrown by boys ($M = 8.4$ m, $SD = 2.4$ m), a finding in exact agreement with Hardin and Garcia (1982). However, when a linear composite of biological variables (joint diameters, shoulder/hip ratio, and skinfolds) was taken into account, girls' predicted performance became 69% that of boys.

When 26 of these children (13 girls and 13 boys) were tested more than 3 years later (Nelson et al., 1991), girls' ($M = 8.8$ m, $SD = 1.9$) performance was only 47% that of boys ($M = 18.7$ m, $SD = 4.5$). The only biological variable that was predictive of performance for the boys at 9 years of age was arm muscle, while a composite of variables related to size (weight, skinfolds, joint diameters, arm muscle, leg muscle, and body mass index) was predictive for girls.

Throwing form was evaluated in both studies (Nelson et al., 1986; Nelson et al., 1991). The form ratings showed boys with better form than girls at 5 years of age; however, by 9 years of age the girls had improved their form very little while boys topped out on the rating scale. Taken together with the fact that biological variables related to size were the significant predictors of throwing performance for 9-year-old girls, it seems likely that girls are only throwing farther as a result of increased size, with little change in throwing mechanics. Boys seem to throw farther because they become larger, but they also improve the mechanics of the throwing motion.

Environment

What are reasons that girls might not improve the mechanics of throwing over the period of childhood and adolescence? During the preschool years, parents tend to emphasize the development of gross motor skills more in boys than in girls (Maccoby & Jacklin, 1974). For example, parents, peers, teachers, and coaches all expect boys and girls to perform many motor tasks differently (Sherif & Rattray, 1976), including throwing. Girls are not encouraged to become better at throwing. There is an often-heard phrase that clearly indicates this and brings to mind an exact movement pattern: "Throws like a girl."

Practice. Boys not only participate in more baseball activities than girls but they also recall practicing overhand throwing more than girls (Halverson, Roberton, & Langendorfer, 1982). In fact, in training studies the gender differences in throwing performance are not reduced (Dusenberry, 1952; Halverson, Roberton, Safrit, & Roberts, 1977). Effects that are robust to training seem more likely to reflect a biological influence.

Antiquity of Human Throwing

Overhand throwing is an important motor behavior in human society. Throwing may also have played an important role in human evolution. In this section we overview this role with attention to throwing in our closest relatives, chimpanzees, as well as throwing in early humans; we then suggest how human evolution might have played a role in the development of observed gender differences in throwing.

Throwing by Nonhuman Primates

Chimpanzees throw sticks, branches, stones, and rocks as part of their display during aggressive encounters with other chimpanzees, baboons, humans, and other species (Goodall, 1986). Goodall (1970) describes both underhand and overarm throwing in the chimpanzees at Gombe, and disagrees with Kortlandt's (1967) statement that overhand throwing is not part of the natural behavioral inventory of chimpanzees. Kortlandt (1972) reports only underhand throwing and notes that the motor patterns and aim are more developed among savanna chimpanzees than in the forest-dwelling groups he observed.

Most chimpanzee throwing observed by Sugiyama and Koman (1979) is with an underhand pattern, but they report two cases of a sidearm pattern, and six of overarm, the latter by infant and juvenile males and an adolescent female. In some cases the pattern of chimpanzee throwing recalls that of human Frisbee throwing, in which the object is held between the thumb and the side of the flexed index finger and is not encumbered by the long fingers (personal observation).

The objects may be aimed at specific targets (Goodall, 1986; Sugiyama & Koman, 1979), but Goodall has noted that when they are aimed they frequently miss their target. However, she has also observed for some chimpanzees that accuracy in hitting targets improves with the frequency of throwing. Goodall (1970) suggests that success of accidental throwing, which occurs occasionally when chimpanzees release objects from the hand when the arm is waved about in aggressive encounters, may provide incentive to repeat the throwing behavior.

Both male and female pygmy chimpanzees (Jordan, 1982) and common chimpanzees (Goodall, 1986; Sugiyama & Koman, 1979) are reported to throw. Not all of them throw, and only a few of those that do throw were observed to do so frequently. Goodall did find clear-cut differences between adult males and females in the frequency of aimed throwing.

Over a period of 6 years, during which throwing bouts were recorded at Gombe, 5 of 7 adult males threw at least twice whereas only 3 of 12 females threw at all. No adult female threw more than five times in a given year, but one adult male threw more than 50 times. (Goodall, 1970, does note, however, that one female at Gombe did become an expert thrower.) Immature males also throw more than immature females (Goodall, 1986). Sugiyama and Koman (1979) also report a higher frequency of throwing among males.

Throwing occurs during play by immature chimpanzees. Sugiyama and Koman (1979) describe throwing by adolescent and juvenile animals among themselves, in situations that are not part of aggressive display behaviors, and Goodall (1986) reports aggressive play in which throwing is directed toward young baboons.

Evidence for Early Human Throwing

Several authors have speculated that the throwing of objects in displays may have been a factor in the origin of human tool use for protection of the group and also for foraging (Goodall, 1968; Hall, 1963; Kortlandt & Kooij, 1963; Lancaster, 1968; Washburn & Jay, 1967). Since it is a behavior observed in our closest relatives, it is reasonable to assume that it was within the potential range of behavior of human ancestors as they evolved in adaptation to feeding and moving about primarily on the ground.

Calvin (1983b) and Darlington (1975) have emphasized the advantage that this behavior provides in inflicting damage at a distance, when a modern human throws with skill. The degree of skill is a function of several interrelated features of the human hand, locomotor apparatus, and brain (Marzke 1983, 1986, in press).

There are three circumstances in which forceful, accurate aimed throwing might have enhanced protective and foraging behavior of early humans. First, it should have positively influenced the deterring effect of displays, if the missiles consistently hit the intruders and inflected injury. Second, if humans incorporated scavenging into their foraging behavior, accurate and forceful throwing should have contributed to their ability to displace other scavenging species from a carcass. Third, hunting of game would have become more effective, and less dangerous to humans, as their ability to throw forcefully and accurately allowed them to stun small prey with stones, and eventually to inflict greater damage at greater distances as the tools thrown became more sophisticated.

There is considerable debate, however, as to whether scavenging and hunting were indeed significant elements of early human foraging behavior, and as to when hunting might have become a behavior frequent and crucial enough to have been a factor in the evolution of features in the human hand, locomotor apparatus, and brain.

Morphology of Modern Human Skilled Throwing

Forceful throwing of missiles with speed and accuracy requires recruitment of the full anatomical link system involving the feet, ankles, legs, thighs, trunk, arm, forearm, wrist, and hand. A comparison of this system between apes and humans reveals differences that probably affect the ability of an ape to apply and integrate these links as effectively as humans in throwing (Marzke 1983, 1986, in press). Two fundamental elements of aimed throwing are controlled rotation of the trunk and controlled release of the missile.

Initial trunk rotation away from the direction of the throw carries the arm backward and increases the distance over which the arm will accelerate. This is followed by trunk rotation in the direction of the throw, which contributes to the acceleration of the missile through the trunk and arm segments. Then comes braking of trunk rotation in the direction of the throw as the arm approaches the level of the ear.

This braking of the trunk segment results in further acceleration of the arm segments prior to release of the missile (Marzke, Longhill, & Rasmussen, 1988). For example, Figure 5 (revised from Figure 2 in Marzke et al., 1988) shows the right gluteus maximus muscle firing (EMG) as the trunk begins to rotate in the direction of the throw. The left gluteus maximus muscle is contracting as the trunk stops rotation, producing maximal arm acceleration. Notice the much quicker

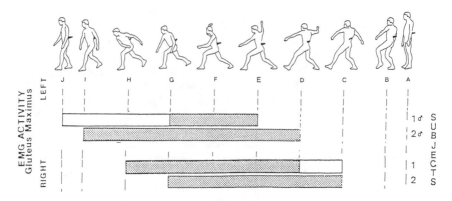

Figure 5 — Gluteus maximus muscle EMG firing patterns in an expert and a novice thrower. From Marzke, Longhill, and Rasmussen (1988, p. 522). Copyright 1988 by Wiley-Liss. Reprinted with permission.

"turn-on, turn-off" firing pattern of the left gluteus maximus in Subject 1, an expert in throwing, as compared to Subject 2, a novice.

In apes, the potential for applying the rotation and leverage of the trunk to the acceleration of a missile is limited by (a) the disproportionate distribution of weight superior and anterior to the hip joints and (b) the lack of a muscle acting on the hip joint that has the force and mechanical advantage to control the movements of the heavy upper trunk and forelimbs.

In humans, the center of mass lies at the level of the second sacral vertebra, above and between the hip joints, so that balance of the upper body on the legs and feet requires less extensive muscle recruitment. In addition, a large gluteus maximus muscle attaches high on the pelvis, well superior to the hip joint, where it is able not only to resist forward collapse of the trunk as forelimb momentum increases but also to initiate and halt trunk rotation in a manner that enhances the movement of the arm. In apes this muscle is relatively small and attaches only to the caudal vertebrae, sacrum, and projecting ischium.

Controlled release of the missile is achieved in humans by maneuvering the missile with the palmar friction surfaces of the long thumb and short fingers. This activity of course involves coordination by the brain of the elements within the hand and of the hand and eyes.

Differences between humans and apes in the relative proportions of the thumb and fingers (Marzke, 1983, in press), and in the relative size of the cortical areas controlling the hand (Penfield & Rasmussen; Woolsey & Settlage, cited in Washburn, 1959), undoubtedly constrain the control with which apes are able to strike a target, using the overhand throwing pattern of humans. Calvin (1983a) and Marshack (1984a,b) have speculated in a very general way on the nature of changes in brain circuitry that might have evolved with evolution of the hand and tool use in humans.

Skilled Throwing in Early Humans

Given these apparent differences between apes and humans in the potential for skilled throwing with the modern human overhand pattern, is it possible to infer from morphology of fossil human ancestors their potential for throwing forcefully and accurately with speed? Skeletal remains of the earliest members of our family, Hominidae, dating back at least 3 million years, throw (pun intended) interesting light on this question.

The structure of the pelvis and the relative proportions of the limbs in the skeleton of *Australopithecus afarensis* indicate that the center of mass was located more inferiorly than in apes, probably permitting better balance of the upper body on the hindlimbs (Jungers & Stern, 1983). A marking on the pelvis of *Australopithecus africanus* from Makapan indicates that the gluteus maximus muscle attached to the ilium (Dart, 1949), although the attachment may not have been fully developed (Stern, 1972).

It is evident, then, that soon after our divergence from the line leading to modern chimpanzees and gorillas, there were features in early hominids that might have enhanced the use of the trunk as leverage in throwing. It is also interesting to note that the thumb was longer relative to the fingers in *Australopithecus afarensis* than it is in apes (Marzke, 1983), and that the hand appears to have been capable of controlling objects by the palmar friction surfaces of the thumb, index, and third fingers, just as modern humans maneuver baseballs in the "three-jawed chuck" grip (Marzke, 1983).

These features are part of a morphological mosaic in early hominids, which includes a number of ape-like elements. The brains of these species were approximately the size of the brains of apes, relative to body size. The fingers and toes were somewhat curved and appear to have been used in climbing (Marzke, 1983; Stern & Susman, 1983).

It is difficult to speculate as to how effectively the full link system might have functioned in throwing, since the elements combined modern human-like features with modern ape-like features and formed a whole that probably functioned in a way not observed in any living species. However, several features that seem to enhance modern human skillful throwing appeared together early in our evolution.

One cannot necessarily argue that the features evolved exclusively in adaptation in throwing, or that throwing was crucial to early human survival. But note that (a) throwing is a characteristic element of behavior in our closest living relative, the chimpanzee, (b) the Australopithecines had several morphological features that together should have enhanced their ability to use this throwing behavior to greater advantage than is generally characteristic of chimpanzees, and (c) throwing in historical times has been widespread and effective in both defensive behavior and predation (Isaac, 1987).

In this context the Australopithecine evidence is suggestive of an early stage in human evolution, in which a behavior that previously had lacked an interrelated set of specialized morphological correlates was becoming habitual and successful enough to have focused selection on features that later would occur together frequently in modern humans.

Historical Evidence for the Importance of Throwing

Isaac (1987) has strengthened the argument for a significant role of throwing in the early stages of hominid evolution by drawing attention to reports in the ethnographic and historical literature of extremely skillful and effective throwing by people without well-developed technologies, in defensive encounters and during hunting of small and even relatively large game. One frequently sees this behavior even today, for instance when unarmed people are subjected to gunfire or tear gas. The importance of Isaac's review is her demonstration of the extraordinary force and accuracy with which stones, thrown skillfully by modern humans, hit their targets.

This evidence brackets, with the nonhuman primate evidence of throwing in aggressive display, the fossil evidence of evolution in neural and musculoskeletal features that facilitate skillful throwing. As Isaac makes clear, these three lines of evidence for the importance of throwing in human evolution are all circumstantial, but yet together they are inherently consistent.

Evidence of Gender Differences in Throwing

Still more tenuous, but potentially compelling, are three lines of evidence for considerable antiquity of gender differences in throwing: (a) the findings in contemporary samples of human children and adults of differences in throwing pattern, outlined above, (b) brief references in the literature to a higher frequency of throwing among male chimpanzees (Goodall, 1986; Sugiyama & Koman, 1979), and (c) the finding by Isaac (1987, p. 15) that "all historical instances so far quoted relate to throwing by males, with the honourable exception of the Australian Aborigines."

There is no doubt that differences in the frequency with which male and female chimpanzees and humans throw, and perhaps also in some elements of throwing patterns in humans, may be attributed to gender differences in socialization. However, these differences in social behavior are more accessible to study than potential differences in morphological and neurophysiological correlates of throwing, and the possibility that the latter differences exist should be explored.

Studying the Development of Gender Differences in Throwing

If we wish to determine factors that are related to the development of gender differences in throwing, as well as whether these differences may have developed through evolutionary processes, we must study the throwing pattern and its neuromuscular control in detail. We cannot make sound scientific decisions from qualitative assessments. The qualitative assessments we have developed are quite useful for teachers and coaches; they allow a movement analysis with the eye and a subsequent correction. However, qualitative movement analysis techniques are not useful for attributing underlying mechanisms and causes.

We must use a combination of techniques such as high-speed video that can be digitized to total body models, EMG recordings of appropriate muscle groups, and ground reaction forces in order to accurately measure the movement characteristics and test hypotheses about the evolution of throwing. These techniques will allow us to determine

- whether expert males and females use the same throwing pattern supported by the same muscle groups, organized in the same manner;
- the developmental patterns of boys and girls as they progress toward throwing expertise and mature models;
- whether intense training programs can alter the pattern of female throwing;

- whether carrying an object (simulating an infant) in one arm by males and females produces similar throwing characteristics; and
- whether our closest primate relatives (chimpanzees) use overhand throwing patterns similar to humans and whether male and female chimpanzees use the same pattern.

Suggestions About the Developmental Aspects of Sport Performance

Your first question might be, Are there any applications? We believe so. For example, as you evaluate our report here about throwing in expert males and females, it becomes obvious that we know very little about a movement pattern that underlies some of the most important sports in our culture and that may have played an important role in human evolution.

1. Are the expert male and female throwing patterns really different, as our small sample of data suggest? Have we pinpointed the important differences, or are there others? Does EMG activity differ in the major muscle groups supporting trunk rotation and arm action? How are the ground reaction forces associated with this movement pattern? Do ground reaction forces differ by gender in their relation to throwing patterns?

2. If any of the characteristics listed above really differ in male and female experts, what are the implications for instruction and training of children, adults, novices, and experts? For instance, have we been attempting to train women to throw like men, when in fact training them to use the female throwing pattern more efficiently would result in better performance?

3. Do any of the characteristics in Item 1 relate to the high injury rate often associated with overhand throwing (e.g., rotator cuff, elbow)?

In summary, gender differences in throwing are much larger and much sooner in development than other motor skills. This has led us to consider the question of whether the overhand throwing pattern in female and male experts is similar or different. Given some evidence that patterns may differ, might there be a human evolution explanation for the gender differences? Circumstantial evidence from antiquity suggests a potential connection.

References

Calvin, W.H. (1982). Did throwing stones shape hominid brain evolution? *Ethology and Sociobiology*, **3**, 115-124.

Calvin, W.H. (1983a). A stone's throw and its launch window: Timing precision and its implications for language and hominid brains. *Journal of Theoretical Biology*, **104**, 121-135.

Calvin, W.H. (1983b). *The throwing madonna*. New York: McGraw Hill.

Darlington, P.J. Jr. (1975). Group selection, altruism, reinforcement, and throwing in human evolution. *Proceedings of the National Academy of Sciences*, **72**, 3748-3752.

Dart, R.A. (1949). Innominate fragments of *Australopithecus prometheus*. American *Journal of Physical Anthropology*, **7**, 301-336.

Dusenberry, L.M. (1952). A study of the effects of training in ball throwing by children ages three to seven. *Research Quarterly*, **23**, 9-14.

Eaton, W.O., & Enns, L.R. (1986). Sex differences in human motor activity level. *Psychological Bulletin*, **100**, 19-28.

Goodall, J. (1968). The behaviour of free-living chimpanzees in the Gombe Stream Reserve. *Animal Behaviour Monographs*, **1**, 161-311.

Goodall, J. (1970). Tool-using in primates and other vertebrates. In D. Lehrman, R. Hinde, & E. Shaw (Eds.), *Advances in the study of behavior* (Vol. 3, pp. 195-249). New York: Academic Press.

Goodall, J. (1986). *The chimpanzees of Gombe: Patterns of behavior*. Cambridge: Harvard University Press.

Hall, K.R.L. (1963). Tool-using performances as indicators of behavioral adaptability. *Current Anthropology*, **4**, 479-494.

Halverson, L.E., Roberton, M.A., & Langendorfer, S. (1982). Development of the overarm throw: Movement and ball velocity changes by seventh grade. *Research Quarterly for Exercise and Sport*, **53**, 198-205.

Halverson, L.E., Roberton, M.A., Safrit, M.J., & Roberts, T.W. (1977). Effect of guided practice on overhand throw ball velocities of kindergarten children. *Research Quarterly*, **48**, 311-318.

Hardin, D., & Garcia, M. (1982). Diagonostic performance tests for elementary children (grades 1–4). *Journal of Physical Education, Recreation and Dance*, **53**(2), 48.

Isaac, B. (1987). Throwing and human evolution. *The African Archaeological Review*, **5**, 3-17.

Jordan, C. (1982). Object manipulation and tool-use in captive pygmy chimpanzees (*Pan paniscus*). *Journal of Human Evolution*, **11**, 35-39.

Jungers, W.L., & Stern, J.T. (1983). Body proportions, skeletal allometry and locomotion in the Hadar hominids: A reply to Wolpoff. *Journal of Human Evolution*, **12**, 673-684.

Kortlandt, A. (1967). Handgebrauch bei freilebenden Schimpansen [Use of the hand by free-living chimpanzees]. In B. Rensch (Ed.), *Handgebrauch und verstandigung bei affen und fruhmenschen* (pp. 59-102). Bern and Stuttgart: Huber.

Kortlandt, A. (1972). *New perspectives on ape and human evolution*. Amsterdam: Stichting Voor Psychobiologie.

Kortlandt, A., & Kooij, M. (1963). Protohominid behaviour in primates. *Symposia of the Zoological Society of London*, **10**, 61-88.

Lancaster, J.B. (1968). On the evolution of tool-using behavior. *American Anthropologist*, **70**, 56-66.

Maccoby, E.E., & Jacklin, C.N. (1974). *The psychology of sex differences*. Stanford, CA: Stanford University Press.

Marshack, A. (1984a). *Hierarchical evolution of the human capacity: The Paleolithic evidence* (James Arthur Lecture). New York: American Museum of Natural History.

Marshack, A. (1984b). The ecology and brain of two-handed bipedalism: An analytic, cognitive, and evolutionary assessment. In H.L. Roitblat, T.G. Bever, & H.S. Terrace (Eds.), *Animal cognition* (pp. 491-511). Hillsdale, NJ: Erlbaum.

Marzke, M.W. (in press). Evolution of the hand and bipedality. In A. Lock & C. Peters (Eds.), *Handbook of human symbolic evolution*. Oxford: Oxford University Press.

Marzke, M.W. (1983). Joint functions and grips of the *Australopithecus afarensis* hand, with special reference to the region of the capitate. *Journal of Human Evolution, 12,* 197-211.

Marzke, M.W. (1986). Tool use and the evolution of hominid hands and bipedality. In J.G. Else & P.C. Lee (Eds.), *Proceedings of the Tenth Congress of the International Primatological Society* (Vol. 1, pp. 203-209). London: Cambridge University Press.

Marzke, M.W., Longhill, J.M., & Rasmussen, S.A. (1988). Gluteus maximus muscle function and the origin of hominid bipedality. *American Journal of Physical Anthropology, 77,* 519-528.

Nelson, K.R., Thomas, J.R., & Nelson, J.K. (1991). Longitudinal changes in throwing performance: Gender differences. *Research Quarterly for Exercise and Sport, 62,* 105-108.

Nelson, J.K., Thomas, J.R., Nelson, K.R., & Abraham, P.C. (1986). Gender differences in children's throwing performance: Biology and environment. *Research Quarterly for Exercise and Sport, 57,* 280-287.

Rippee, N.E., Pangrazi, R.P., Corbin, C.B., Borsdorf, L., Petersen, B., & Pangrazi, D. (1991). Throwing profiles of first and fourth grade boys and girls. *The Physical Educator, 47,* 180-185.

Roberton, M.A. (1982). Describing stages within and across motor tasks. In J.A.S. Kelso & J.E. Clark (Eds.), *The development of movement control and co-ordination* (pp. 293-307). New York: Wiley & Sons.

Roberton, M.A. (1984). Changing motor patterns during childhood. In J.R. Thomas (Ed.), *Motor development during childhood and adolescence* (pp. 48-90). Minneapolis: Burgess.

Seefeldt, V., & Haubenstricker, J. (1982). Patterns, phases, or stages: An analytical model for the study of developmental movement. In J.A.S. Kelso & J.E. Clark (Eds.), *The development of movement control and co-ordination* (pp. 309-318). New York: Wiley & Sons.

Sherif, C.W., & Rattray, G.D. (1976). Psychological development and activity in middle childhood. In J.G. Albinson & G.M. Andrew (Eds.), *Child in sport and physical activity* (pp. 97-132). Baltimore: University Park Press.

Smoll, F.L., & Schutz, R.W. (1990). Quantifying gender differences in physical performance: A developmental perspective. *Developmental Psychology, 26,* 360-369.

Stern, J.T. (1972). Anatomical and functional specializations of the human gluteus maximus. *American Journal of Physical Anthropology, 36,* 315-340.

Stern, J.T., & Susman, R.L. (1983). The locomotor anatomy of *Australopithecus afarensis*. *American Journal of Physical Anthropology, 60,* 279-317.

Sugiyama, Y., & Koman, J. (1979). Tool-using and -making behavior in wild chimpanzees at Bossou, Guinea. *Primates, 20,* 513-524.

Thomas, J.R., & French, K.E. (1985). Gender differences across age in motor performance: A meta-analysis. *Psychological Bulletin*, **98**, 260-282.

Thomas, J.R., & Thomas, K.T. (1988). Development of gender differences in physical activity. *Quest*, **40**, 219-229.

Thomas, J.R., Thomas, K.T., & Gallagher, J.D. (in press). Developmental considerations in skill acquisition. In R.N. Singer et al. (Eds.), *Handbook on research in sport psychology*. New York: Macmillan.

Washburn, S.L. (1959). Speculations on the interrelations of the history of tools and biological evolution. In J.N. Spuhler (Ed.), *The evolution of man's capacity for culture* (pp. 21-31). Detroit: Wayne State University Press.

Washburn, S.L., & Jay, P. (1967). More on tool-use among primates. *Current Anthropology*, **8**, 253-254.

Gender Differences in Throwing: Evolutionary Evidence or More Monkey Business? A Reaction to Thomas and Marzke

Michael G. Wade
University of Minnesota

I would like first to thank the Academy and President-elect Bob Christina for inviting me to react to the Thomas and Marzke paper entitled "The Development of Gender Differences in Throwing: Is Human Evolution a Factor?"

The essential point that Thomas and Marzke would wish to make in their provocative paper is that gender differences in throwing, and the persistence and size of this difference (Thomas & French, 1985), are such that they require description beyond the usual standard accounts. The four points they make are as follows:

1. Biomechanical analysis of gender differences has been insufficient, and there is a need to examine more closely the difference between novice throwers and experts.
2. The evidence from evolutionary biology suggests that throwing may well be a special case of motor skill activity and that there are deeper and more important developmental reasons for the observed gender differences.
3. These differences are, to use their term, "hard wired."
4. There are implications in the gender differences in throwing that have implications for sport performance.

From the outset I do not find the arguments presented by Thomas and Marzke particularly compelling. Thus I cannot share their enthusiasm for making the differences in this skill activity special.

The first question I would ask is, What is so special about gender differences in throwing? Their rationale seems to rely on the findings reported in Thomas and French's 1985 meta-analysis, which reports that the performance difference (effect size) in throwing between males and females is larger than that observed for other motor skills. This conclusion is insufficient to go searching for a cause and effect relationship in gender differences in throwing.

Thomas and Marzke would have us believe that in addition to the meta-analysis data there is cross-cultural evidence of performance stability for throwing as a task, and that training effects appear not to reduce gender differences over time. Further, they raise the issue from earlier work that lateralization, brain size, and redundancy may also be issues that single out throwing as a special candidate in motor performance.

The difference between males and females in throwing is not a new issue to the study of gender and physical activity. In 1938 at this very meeting, held that year in Atlanta, Monica Wild of the State Teacher's College in Cedar Falls, Iowa, presented an interesting paper (Wild, 1938) that sought to determine differences in the pattern (kinematics) of throwing and its relationship to development in children. Wild employed a relatively crude protocol, yet she produced a sophisticated paper that analyzed initial velocities of forceful overhand throwing in young children between the ages of 2 and 7 years.

The subjects were selected in such a way that she was able to test the possible gender differences in both the manner (style) of throwing and the distance thrown. She reported differences between boys and girls in throwing velocity, and also in the horizontal path and the point of release in vigorous overhand throwing. Wild concluded with some quite sophisticated insights:

> maturational factors are believed to be operative as the basic type patterns of throwing develop; learning, particularly after six years, greatly influences the skill pattern, individuating out of and upon the basic growth stage; it may be the factor accountable for differences in performance, especially those so evident between the sexes. (p. 24)

She went on to note, "The genetic history of the hard overhand throw and the panorama of change in the movement and timing features of successive stages in throwing behavior afford a valuable background for the solution of problems arising in respect to the throwing, play and games of children" (p. 24). Wild identified some of the elements and issues raised by Thomas and Marzke in their paper, and included data to describe some of these differences in terms of the kinetics of throwing.

A more recent paper by Leme and Shambes (1978) sought to determine and describe immature throwing patterns in normal women. They employed cinemetagraphic techniques to collect data and expanded upon Wild's 1938 paper in attempting to better understand the developmental stages of throwing in children. Comparing adults (male and female) with children, Leme and Shambes concluded that adults exhibit immature throwing patterns which appeared directly analogous to the more primitive stages identified in young children.

They concluded that the immature motor patterns recorded in women may be attributed to motivational, social, or cultural reasons as well as biological factors. Their data implied that many adults have not progressed beyond a particular stage of throwing. Thus, immature throwing patterns in women should not be considered incorrect but rather should be viewed as manifestations of what they call "early inherent motor patterns," which are executed correctly for that particular stage.

The papers by Wild (1938) and by Leme and Shambes (1978) contain the kind of biomechanical data called for by Thomas and Marzke to analyze the kinematics of the overarm throw. This was an issue we addressed in our laboratory (Wade & Hamill, 1984) when we recorded young children and adults (college students) performing the overarm throw using their preferred hand and, in the case of the adults, their nonpreferred hand, to compare the kinematic profiles of the mature throwers with those of the young children. We employed Wild's 1938 classification system to place subjects into Stages 1, 3, and 5 of throwing style.

The data are presented in Figure 1, and what we observed was a similarity in the kinematic profiles of the young children's throwing (recorded as Stages 1 and 3) and the adult throwing, labeled Stage 5. The differences are expressed in the ordinate values (vertical displacement) and the relative motion of wrist, elbow, and shoulder between Stage 1 and Stage 5. In addition, the range of the horizontal displacement (abscissa) values were different for Stages 1 and 5. Note that the nonpreferred throwing hand of the mature thrower, labeled "Stage 5, nonpreferred," is essentially the same profile as that of the Stage 3 child throwing with a preferred hand.

The absolute values of vertical and horizontal displacement are different but the throwing pattern is the same. If one considers the degrees of freedom involved in the shoulder, arm, and wrist joint system for recording the kinematics of the overarm throw, this is not surprising. In fact, I would argue that kinematic analysis of the throwing arm will reveal little about gender differences between throwers.

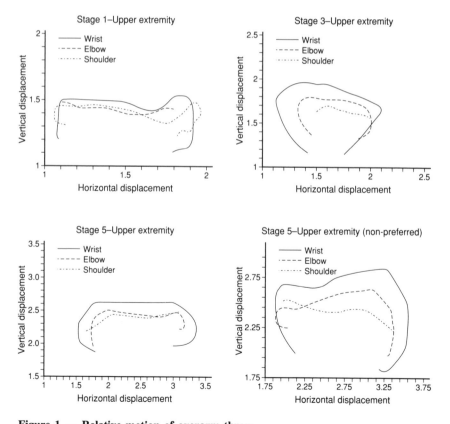

Figure 1 — Relative motion of overarm throw.

The secret of gender differences in throwing is less obvious in the kinematic patterns of the upper arm, which is a highly constrained special purpose device that most likely resides in the temporal (coordinated) relationship between the upper arm and the power and speed generated from the trunk and lower limbs. The angular displacement between hip and shoulder acting together to generate peak velocity to the arm and hand would seem a better candidate to account for gender differences in this activity.

In my judgment, EMG and ground reaction force data may well help clarify this gender related issue. Throwing differences are best explained by the power generated by the trunk and lower limbs from the more mesomorphic content of the male physique compared with that of the female. This is reflected in a capacity to generate higher levels of peak velocity and acceleration, reflected in some of the descriptive data presented by Thomas and Marzke.

It is not surprising then that males are favored in this kind of activity, simply because they are bigger, stronger, and more powerful. Size as a biological entity has been, and remains an important and interesting contributor to variability in motor performance (McMahon, 1975).

In briefly examining evolutionary biology and its influence in producing gender differences of the kind that are the focus of the Thomas and Marzke paper, a brief review of what in biology is called "life history" and the techniques and procedures referred to as allometry is required. Life history implicates the evolutionary differences of power reflected in such motor activities as running, jumping, and throwing.

If we agree that throwing is the most skillful of these activities, the allometric considerations for such an activity as overhand throwing seek a better understanding and a recognition that organisms are adapted by natural selection to both their physical and biological environments. Allometry examines the effects of size on such variables as growth rate, age at first reproduction, food intake, and energy requirements. This body of knowledge and any theories growing out of it are known generally as life history.

Gender differences are broadly associated with the domain that considers such variables as the mean or average daily metabolic rate, the energy assimilation, and the relationship of those factors to body weight. Generally speaking, allometric coefficients that relate mean daily metabolic rate to body weight (W) have a value of $W^{.65-.75}$ and to energy assimilation of $W^{.67}$ across a wide range of species from fish to primates.

The differences in size between males and females rest primarily on the question of the energy available for reproduction versus other energy requirements. Larger species invest relatively less time and energy in their offspring. It has been concluded that while females can be up to 1,000 times heavier than males, males are never more than 8 times heavier than females (Reiss, 1989). Thus, males can only devote between 3 and 10% of their time in attempting reproduction, and larger species show considerable degrees of sexual dimorphism, although there are some exceptions.

While allometry is not as precise as, for example, Mendel's law of genetics, size plays a significant role in a species' investment in offspring and the duration of parental investment. Critical are such variables as weight of offspring versus the weight and duration of parental investment, the effects of litter size on the mother and offspring, the shape of the offspring fitness curves to parental invest-ment, and the forces operating on the timing of the birth when parental invest-ment is to continue after birth. In addition, energy consequences to the parent of offspring are important when the offspring is carried postnatally (one of the issues alluded to in the Thomas and Marzke paper).

The effects of predatation on a larger mammal's time to reach reproduc-tive maturity and the energy reserves when having to deal with seasonal environ-ments are disadvantageous to large animals. What all this says is that allometric variables have significant implications for the biological basis of differences between the sexes (Wade & Berg, in press). Certainly the range of these differ-ences should not be surprising when looked at on some absolute scale of size.

While it is important to consider the influence of evolutionary biology in all physical and biological environments, there are other issues that must be kept in mind when we attempt to make cross-species comparisons between humans and other primates. This is another important cornerstone on which Thomas and Marzke build their case. First, it should be remembered that evolutionary change is not necessarily linear and not directed toward any particular adaptation. The pathway of speciation is perhaps better depicted as the ''bushing out'' of the twigs that form the limbs of the evolutionary tree, which itself is made up of a main trunk and relatively few major limbs. It is the bushing out of the twigs rather than the branches of the major limbs that is significant.

Second, while evolutionary changes may be viewed as changes in the gene pools of various populations, these changes should be viewed partly in terms of habitat (environmental changes). Thus, when comparing humans with other pri-mates, it is important to keep in mind that the human twig grew from the primate branch and to view this in the context of the possible habitat conditions that were associated with this event. Further, while humans and chimpanzees might share a common ancestry and may, from Thomas and Marzke's point of view, arguably be our ''closest cousins,'' it should be remembered that they split from each other 6,000,000 years ago!

There is evidence that, while lateralization (right-hand dominance) is record-ed reliably in humans and gorillas (Schaller, 1963), no such data exist among the chimpanzees (pongo), and in fact what data are available suggest that they are closer to being ambidextrous in their observed motor activities (Finch, 1941). The human brain is distinct from other primate brains and began to evolve millions of years after its evolutionary split from the chimpanzee. Thus it should come as no surprise if there are differences in brain architecture and functioning between humans and chimps, even though both species may well share 99% of their DNA.

Looking for behavior homologues between chimpanzees and humans, especially when complex (cortically mediated) functions are involved, may well be an unproductive enterprise. Further, it should be noted that brain changes between chimpanzees and humans were likely initiated and supported by habitat changes—from heavily forested areas (where chimps resided) to the savanna (where humans resided)—that placed different pressures on both the accompany-ing and developing behaviors for survival.

We must examine with a more critical eye the ''throwing'' behavior that has been exhibited by the chimpanzees. Certainly it can be argued that throwing behavior is more effective in open savanna habitats than in the forested areas, especially the kind that is target directed and requires critical power in order to disable or kill a prey. Given this simple fact, it would be surprising if comparisons between chimpanzees and humans in throwing would produce any interesting insights into the evolution of throwing.

Of more value would be to conduct comparative studies, that is, developmental studies (different ages and experiences) of individuals in different cultures. A key to determining the possible gender differences in throwing may be found in cross-cultural studies within the human population rather than comparing humans with other primates.

Target-directed throwing probably served hunting purposes for humans and more likely display (reproductive) purposes for the chimps. For the economic purposes of hunting, we would see an evolving or perfected throwing behavior in that morph of the sexually dimorphic species that chose to hunt prey for survival. This morph would be male, as contrasted with the female who bore and cared for the young (reproductive) and gathered (economic). Comparative studies of males and females more likely accounts for such evolutionary changes.

While there is a need to go beyond purely descriptive anthropological data and to tackle some of the biologically based allometric issues that investigate the relationship between the effects of size and gender differences, there are, as I have outlined above, some inherent problems in making such comparisons. We simply cannot ignore the issue of sociocultural factors that have played a critical role in all behavior that shows differences between males and females.

In this sense we are then revisiting the old nature/nurture problem. I am not convinced that the Thomas and Marzke paper provides a convincing case to suggest that the differences in overarm throwing are unique and compelling beyond a wide range of gender differences in a variety of physical and biological contexts.

Finally, there is the question of the methodology: the meta-analysis of Thomas and French (1985) and the seemingly conflicting evidence of that reported by Smoll and Schutz (1990) in a study that was better controlled. Smoll and Schutz employed multivariate techniques in determining gender differences in physical performance. They concluded that childhood gender differences are substantially influenced by anthropometric variables, with approximately 50% of between-gender variance being accounted for by fatness alone, and suggested that with advancing age, gender differences may become increasingly more a function of environmental factors.

Certainly Smoll and Schutz's conclusions fit with the broad-based life history data that are available on many species in the animal kingdom but do not represent a solid body of knowledge as it relates to the motor development of homo sapiens. In addition to raising some fundamental questions about the appropriateness of the evolutionary biological rationale advanced by Thomas and Marzke, there is a methodological question as to the appropriateness of meta-analysis for attributing cause and effect, to build a case for gender differences in overarm throwing.

We must remember that the overarm throw involves perhaps the most complicated and most researched anatomical component of the species, namely the hand. Research on the hand has been the focus of much attention (Connolly & Elliott, 1972; Napier, 1956). All forms of throwing require grasping the implement with the hand, which makes all activities involving reaching and grasping of special interest to kinesiological science. Thus the ability to grasp makes any activity involving the hand task-specific and may well account for differences, not only between males and females within a species (i.e., hand size and the scale of the hand to the implement to be grasped or thrown) but also across species, as can be well demonstrated in Figure 2, which illustrates the anatomy of the hand across three species (pongo, gorilla, and homo).

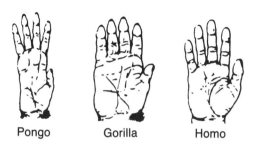

Pongo   Gorilla   Homo

Figure 2 — Hand form for chimpanzee (pongo), gorilla, and homo.

As can be readily appreciated, the hand of the chimpanzee (pongo) is not well adapted for the kind of expert throwing, both in terms of velocity and accuracy claimed by the Thomas and Marzke paper. Certainly it suggests that any throwing behavior by chimpanzees is, as I have suggested along with others before me, focused more on display and reproductive activity than purposeful and intentful activity that would be the case for human throwing in earlier times.

The Thomas and Marzke paper raises some questions and issues that need further research. I hope my reaction has at least given the readership and the Academy pause for reflection and perhaps consideration of some alternative hypotheses and places to look in this ongoing analysis.

Acknowledgment

The author wishes to thank his colleague at Minnesota, Dr. Bill Charlesworth of the Institute of Child Development, for some insightful discussion during the preparation of this reaction paper.

References

Connolly, K.J., & Elliott, J. (1972. The evolution and autogeny of hand function. In N. Burton Jones (Ed.), *Etiological studies of child behavior* (pp. 329-383). Cambridge: Cambridge University Press.

Finch, G. (1941). Chimpanzee handedness. *Science*, **94**, 117-118.

Leme, S.A., & Shambes, G.M. (1978). Immature throwing patterns in normal adult women. *Journal of Human Movement Studies*, **4**, 85-93.

McMahon, T.A. (1975). Using body size to understand the structural design of animals: Quadrupedal motion. *Journal of Applied Physiology*, **39**, 619-627.

Napier, J.R. (1956). The prehensile movements of the human hand. *Journal of Bone and Joint Surgery*, **38B**, 902-913.

Reiss, M.J. (1989). *The allometry of growth and reproduction*. Cambridge: Cambridge University Press.

Schaller, G.B. (1963). *The mountain gorilla: Ecology and behavior*. Chicago: Chicago University Press.

Smoll, F.L., & Schutz, R.W. (1990). Quantifying gender differences in physical performance: A developmental perspective. *Developmental Psychology*, **26**, 361-369.

Thomas, J.R., & French, K.E. (1985). Gender differences across age in motor performance: A meta-analysis. *Psychological Bulletin*, **98**, 260-282.

Wade, M.G., & Berg, W.P. (in press). How to study movement in children. In J. Fagard & P. Wolff (Eds.), *The development of timing control and temporal organization in coordinated action* (*Advances in Psychology Series*). Amsterdam: North Holland Publ.

Wade, M.G., & Hamill, J. (1984, April). *Application of kinesiological methods for enhancing motor skill development in children*. Paper presented at the AAHPERD Research Consortium, Anaheim, CA.

Wild, M. (1938, April). *The behavior pattern of throwing and some observations concerning its course of development in children*. Paper presented at AAHPERD convention, Atlanta.

Beyond Enhancing Performance in Sport: Toward Empowerment and Transformation

George H. Sage
University of Northern Colorado

Bob Christina first contacted me last summer, told me he was developing the 1991 Academy program around the theme "Enhancing Human Performance in Sport," and asked me to make a presentation on this theme from a sociological perspective. I replied by thanking him for the invitation but explained that in recent years a number of us working in the sociology and humanities of physical activity have become increasingly concerned about the cult of performance enhancement that has become such a prominent discourse in kinesiology and some of its allied professions. But, I told him, if he wanted a counterpoint to the theme, I would be willing to do that. Bob responded that he saw no problem with my proposal and would look forward to my presentation. I was delighted with his reply because I saw it as an acknowledgment that various views are legitimate and welcome.

As you are all well aware, concerns have frequently been expressed that our discipline and its allied professions are becoming dominated by the natural science oriented branches of physical activity, and by a positivistic orientation to research, while the social science and humanities of physical activity are being subordinated, and qualitative and hermeneutic methodologies discounted.

Despite disclaimers about such concerns, actions are always more meaningful than words. If we as scholars and practitioners of physical activity are really serious about understanding and appreciating various perspectives about the study of physical activity, if we are *really* going to have an ecumenical working relationship across the various subdisciplines and allied professions, we must be willing to incorporate various views about knowledge production and knowledge dissemination into our scholarship and applied work.

Indeed, questions about knowledge production and dissemination—especially in terms of the question, Knowledge for what ends?—will likely be a continuing issue, because knowledge does not exist apart from how and why it is used and whose interests it represents.

Turning to the theme of this conference, it seems to suggest that the notion of performance enhancement in sport is unproblematic. I want to argue that, as a matter of fact, it is quite problematic. Sport is a value-laden social practice, and meanings in sport, just as with all other cultural practices, are socially constructed. As sociologist Max Weber (1938) said, human beings live in webs of meaning they themselves have spun. Meanings in sport are not immutable or universal; instead they are contested terrain, with social groups constantly struggling for hegemony over its meanings.

What I want to explore in this presentation is the content and context of the discourse of performance enhancement. My focus will be on high performance sport, which encompasses elite youth and adult, college, and professional sports. By "discourse" I mean the ways in which a particular topic or subject area—in this case, performance enhancement in sport—is fashioned, assumptions implicit in its study framed, new knowledge produced, and this knowledge integrated into a field of study.

Discourses are linguistic constructs—the language of topics, the definition of perspectives, portrayal of reality, worldview, but also the buzzwords, specialized vocabulary, and insider's lingo—that become part of the normative understandings which enter into the public expression. Discourses construct reality; and whatever discourses we choose to privilege, we sanction specific human interests and regulate human actions because, once a discourse becomes institutionally privileged, other perspectives are effectively marginalized.

There is a growing critical scholarship directed at discourses of all varieties that support, reinforce, and reproduce dominant versions of social reality in contemporary society. Critical social thought has long been a part of American intellectual tradition in the social sciences and humanities, but in recent years it has been gaining support in the natural sciences as well, primarily as a response to and an interpretation of the turbulence, upheavals, and struggles that have highlighted pervasive political abuses, social contradictions, and economic exploitation and inequalities in America and throughout the world (Shapiro, 1990).

The most salient feature of critical social thought is its focus on analyzing the conditions in which knowledge is created and disseminated. In particular, a critical orientation to knowledge treats "what counts as knowledge" as problematic, thus facilitating analyses into the ways in which knowledge is socially produced, used, and assessed.

In a society in which icons of progress are increasingly drawn from science and technology, critical inquiry seeks to make issues such as how forms of domination and power are maintained and renewed in society *central* to the form and function of science, thereby integrating the purpose of science with that of political engagement and action (Carr & Kemmis, 1986). Science therefore is viewed as fundamentally integrated with the social-political tradition in which it is situated (Popkewitz, 1989). This view, then, disputes the notion that scientific knowledge is objective and value neutral.

Scientific and professional commitment to performance enhancement in sport sounds so noble, so virtuous, so, well, natural. Yet, concealed within this seemingly innocent discourse is a highly selective interpretation of meaning about sport, a scientized, technocratic, instrumentally rational meaning. At the same time, this discourse rests on individualistic meanings about sporting practices; interactional and structural meanings are largely ignored.

From this perspective, sports are abstracted from the institutional and cultural structures and processes in which they are embedded. They are not perceived as socially constructed, historical, and cultural practices that embody political, economic, and ideological interests in which, more often than not, the dominant sectors of society seek to produce knowledge and subjectivities consistent with *their* own agendas. As McKay, Gore, and Kirk (1990) argue, the discourse of performance "entails privileging implicitly and explicitly the values and practices of dominant groups in society" (pp. 66-67).

So the discourse of performance enhancement in sport is not politically neutral, nor is it economically benign, and it certainly is not ideologically harmless. Instead it embodies, albeit tacitly, a sedimented, institutionalized view of the meaning of sport that establishes power over the body and which in turn has significant implications for the organization, form, and content of sport.

Moreover, it contributes to reproducing dominant political, economic, and social relations. Thus the guise of objectivity and neutrality imparted by the discourse of performance enhancement is actually a concrete expression of a larger process of rationalization of bodily practices by intellectual gatekeepers rather than a universal depiction (Foucault, 1977, 1979; Turner, 1982).

From my remarks, I think you can begin to see that a critical agenda for sport seeks to replace objectivist approaches with an analysis that problematizes what counts as legitimate knowledge, and it challenges managerial, efficiency oriented, and technique oriented approaches to the organization and control of sport, replacing them with a social interactive and culturally based critical view.

There is no doubt that throughout history, athletes striving to be the best in their chosen sport have sought ways to improve their performance. But institutional and cultural transformations of the past generation have created unique conditions never before experienced. Over the past 40 years, sport as a commodified industry[1] has spawned a variety of organizations and occupations and it now penetrates every sector of our social lives.

//This industry of mass-produced sports spectacles is "oriented to the commercial and mechanical production of a cult of winning, violent action, physical masculinity, and sensationalized entertainment" (Alt, 1983, p. 97). It seeks to organize sporting events on strict market principles, namely the pursuit of capital accumulation, and it takes for granted that the task of the sport sciences is to discover ways and techniques for systematically producing higher and higher levels of performance in athletes to attract more and more spectators.

As sports, like other cultural practices, have been reconfigured to make them more marketable, an activity "structured by normative rules and imbued with particularized or socially-dominant definitions of the moral purpose of individual achievement and social obligation" (Alt, 1983, p. 93) has been transformed to a dramatization of unadorned commodity relations rather than the satisfaction of individual, personal, and social needs. Whitson (1984) has noted that the growing obsession for record performances has for many "supplanted . . . the less tangible criteria which were once the characteristics of satisfying sporting experiences: style and virtuosity, spontaneity, a 'good game' " (p. 70).

Epistemology and Methodology of Enhanced Performance

A positivistic theory of knowledge guides and shapes the discourse of performance enhancement in sport, and an instrumental rationality undergirds the project

---

[1]The conversion of people, social practices, et cetera, into *things* for sale in the marketplace.

of high performance sport. Positivism, as I use it here, is a mode of thinking and research with a focus on prediction and control and means rather than ends. When this orientation to knowledge is transported unproblematically from the physical and biological sciences into social and cultural settings, timeless and invariant processes in the social universe are postulated similarly to those found in the natural sciences.

As Gibson (1986) notes, just as natural "scientists reify the natural world, seek its laws in order to exercise dominance over it, so, too, positivism reifies the social world [seeking] 'laws' of human conduct in order to exercise more effective control" over it (p. 36). The result "is the manipulation of social relationships, the enthronement of technical means over moral ends, the impoverishment of political discussion, and the support of dominant classes" (Comstock, 1982, p. 373).

Positivist oriented scientists deliberately disengage themselves from conjunctural social issues and withdraw from the salient problems of the rest of the world. They do not ask ethical questions; instead their efforts are given to carefully controlled empirical studies of problems that are normally defined by the state of knowledge in their disciplines rather than by the conditions in society.

Recognition as experts with extraordinary technical competence in a highly specialized but restricted sphere is what they seek (Jacoby, 1987; Lynton, 1987). Adopting a positivistic stance commits them to implicitly accepting "a given set of social arrangements when acting as scientists. They may seek structural change when acting personally, but within a technical understanding of . . . science there can be no scientific legitimation of such efforts" (Bredo & Feinberg, 1982, p. 430).

Positive science is the exemplar for kinesiologists with a preoccupation toward performance enhancement. While there is much that I respect about the work of some of these scientists—and I shamelessly cite them whenever it serves my purposes—there are inherent problems here. Sports, as viewed from this orientation, are conceived of as sophisticated technical pursuits susceptible to "objective treatment." Positivistic reasoning and interest in technical control become translated into hierarchical and bureaucratic control of athletes.

Athletes are viewed as human systems whose effectiveness and efficiency can be enhanced by improving the technology of the system. As professional experts in this system, kinesiologists reflect the basic assumption that methods and techniques of performance enhancement are things that are done for coaches and to athletes, that the expert's task is to define the performance agenda, and the coach's and athlete's tasks as "rational adopters" of innovations, are to apply those findings and techniques (McKay et al., 1990).

A focus on performance enhancement, from a positivistic perspective, tends to endorse an image of sports with enhanced levels of performance as the natural and only "rational" version of sports practice. More important, it leads to an indifference about the interplay of the internal dynamics and social structural role of sports as a cultural practice. Such a tendency makes it difficult to link these internal dynamics to the larger political, economic, and ideological context in which sports take place. As McKay et al. (1990) note,

> Technocratic . . . preoccupation with positivistic methodologies is an outcome of a narrow epistemological perspective that assumes [sporting experience] rests almost exclusively on the understanding of technical phenomena.

. . . It legitimates an ideology of instrumental rationality which is preoccupied with means rather than ends . . . with method and efficiency rather than with purposes. (pp. 56-58)

When a politically neutral and professionally autonomous stance is taken by positive oriented sport scientists, they are deterred from formulating questions such as, Performance enhancement for whom? Performance enhancement for what purposes? But performance enhancement techniques are always used as a means to some end, "and the question of Whose ends? has to be faced up to" (McKay et al., 1990, p. 57).

The major outcome of a positivist model is that it makes it difficult to move beyond producing uncritical renderings about sport and its relation to society so that distorted self-understandings can be clarified and addressed. This makes it difficult to fashion a discourse that historically situates and socially locates sport within its broader societal context. Though sport scientists may not think their work lies within the political, economic, and cultural domain of modern society, this does not exempt it from ideological meaning (Mills, 1959).

The Discourse of Enhanced Performance and Critical Social Thought

Critical social scholarship acknowledges that some contributions made to knowledge by a positivist intellectual orientation are by all means useful; however, the former views the latter's orientation as inadequate because positivism's role, by and large, is one of legitimating social practices "by providing 'objective facts' to justify courses of action. Questions of the values underlying these courses of action" are treated as being beyond the scope of science and are therefore left unexamined (Carr & Kemmis, 1986, p. 132). Moral questions of dominance, control, and power (what for? for whom?) are subordinated from consideration, as the overriding issues of sport are seen primarily as employing new knowledge and technologies to enhance performance (how to?).

To a large extent, the discourse of performance enhancement is an instrument in the growing corporate and government bureaucracies that are committed to high performance sport for profit, in the case of the former, and for systematically improving American sporting achievements in international competition, in the latter. High performance sports have become monuments to "a mechanical quest for efficiency in . . . performance that is indentured to state and commercial sponsorship" (Gruneau, 1979, p. 13).

In fulfilling this function, performance enhancement objectives actually serve to win "consent for a dominant social definition of sport ideally suited to a . . . consumer culture" while at the same time justifying political, economic, and cultural control systems that accept the existing distribution of power in American society as a given (Gruneau, 1989, p. 152).

The linkage of sport scientists to all of this is through their professional expertise. The services of university based scholars have become more marketable with the maturing of capitalism, and this has enlarged the demand and opportunities for money-making. Intellectual work has increasingly become part of the marketplace, with academics marketing their professional expertise for job security, career advancement, and supplemental income (Bok, 1986; Feldman, 1989; Wilshire, 1990).

Because success in sports under the auspices of commercial and state sponsorship is tied directly to outcomes, new opportunities have been created for scientists whose disciplines seem to promise ways of pushing back the frontiers of sports performance. Not surprisingly, they have become part of a growing component of professional experts who pedal their services to corporate and state clients for a fee. They seek to carve out a place for themselves in the industry of high performance sport by offering professional expertise that they alone are able to provide.

Professional services for the sport industry on behalf of performance enhancement, then, have become part of a larger productive process. In this process we witness an alliance between the private sector, the state, and sport science aimed at developing high performing athletes for commercial and political purposes. To a large extent, then, the discourse of performance enhancement in sport aims at the rationalized deployment of material and human resources in pursuit of business, governmental, and professional purposes (Whitson & Macintosh, 1990).

Professional experts always find it difficult to challenge their bureaucratic clients because they are dependent on the good opinion of those clients. Consequently, practitioners of this style of service typically accede to the interests and perspectives of their clients. "To assume this perspective is often in due course to accept it," thus propagating a particular version of meanings, means, and ends in sport (Mills, 1959, p. 101). Inevitably, client dependence undercuts the potential of professional experts as critics.

From all this, one can begin to see the outlines of what types of social relations result from this situation: the dependence of athletes on scientists and professionals who profit from their clients' support. Such a situation leads sport scientists to serve, however unwittingly, the function of reproducing the inequitable social structure and to proceed as if the societal status quo should go unquestioned.

Just as science and technology have been appropriated by dominant economic interests to create new and influential industries, science and technology have also been appropriated to serve commodified sports interests. The emerging industry of so-called sport sciences, whose primary mission seems to be performance enhancement, is committed to searching for the most effective techniques for achieving maximum performance from the programmed body of the athlete.

These scientists attempt to manipulate and control athletes just as physical scientists manipulate objects of the physical world. The rituals and ceremonies of empirical research give their practices legitimacy. Within this system, those who possess scientific knowledge about performance enhancement become the mediators between science and coaches and athletes. Again, we see the type of social relations that emerge, "namely the dependence of the users towards the holders of a single legitimate knowledge" (Harvey, 1986, p. 61).

This science of sport approach offers a pertinent example of Habermas' contention that "for every isolatable cultural area that . . . can be analyzed . . . in terms of presupposed system goals, a new discipline [or science] emerges that explores what is technically possible'' (1970, p. 57). In elaborating on this point, Habermas argued,

> the application of science in technology and the feedback of technical progress to research have become the substance of the world of work. . . . science—to the very extent that it has penetrated professional practice—has estranged itself from humanistic culture. . . . The sciences now transmit a specific capacity: but the capacity for control, which they teach, is not the same capacity for life and action that was to be expected of the scientifically educated and cultivated. (p. 55)

The athlete's body has become an instrument, an object to be worked on, trained, tuned, and manipulated in order to achieve maximum performance. Indeed, high performance sport has increasingly become a project in human engineering whose objective is producing levels of performance with seemingly little understanding, or even interest in, what the consequences may be for the physical, not to mention the personal-social, development of athletes.

John Alt (1983) explains, "like the employee, the athlete is removed from effective control over his[her] athletic labor and his[her] performance is subdivided and monitored by efficiency experts. . . . The similarity of the role of the athlete to that of the employee allows him[her] to perform in a manner conducive to the commercial requirements of the spectacle: to be a winner at all costs" (p. 103). Under the guise of helping athletes, these services actually construct new and increasingly higher performance standards and establish new powers over the body. In this regard, Bruce Kidd (1990) has noted,

> The "competitive mindset" is constructed with the help of the sports [scientists], often without regard to the implications for mature character development and long-term mental health. The athletes' central reality—what sport has come to mean in the day-to-day—is the necessity to perfect themselves to perform at the limits of human physical potential and attempt to surpass those limits. (p. 7)

Coaches, trainers, sport scientists, and even athletes themselves, objectify the athlete's body as if it existed, or the performance it produces existed, separate from the individual (Donnelly, 1990).

Michel Foucault's work (1977) has brought the issue of the discipline of the body and the rise of scientific knowledge to the forefront, and while he does not specifically address contemporary sport, his ideas warrant our reflection in connection with the discourse of performance enhancement. A central theme of Foucault's examination of systematic knowledge is that its growth has been accompanied by an extension of power and control over bodies in social space. For Foucault, scientific advances, while having alleviated much human misery, have not liberated the body from external control; instead they have actually intensified the ways and means of social regulation.

Indeed there does seem to be a manipulative solution for every problem athletes might encounter. If athletes suffer from anxiety, they are taught stress management techniques so they can perform better. If times and distances are not meeting expectations, intensified training regimens are prescribed to improve strength and endurance. Drugs (legal and illegal) and nutritional supplements are administered to enhance performance and elicit sustained training levels that would not be possible without them.[2]

Instead of being grounded in a rejection of the norms of sport, the use of performance enhancing drugs is grounded in an overacceptance and overconformity to those norms. Thus, Ben Johnson has been called a "positive deviant" because he was actually conforming to commonly accepted norms of the discourse of performance enhancement (Coakley, 1989). Under these conditions it is very difficult to draw the line between health and pathology.

I am not implying that athletes, especially those who wish to compete at the highest levels, should not be given the chance to be the very best they can be. I am not denying the importance of seeking ways to improve performance. However, I am suggesting that we need to be the outspoken advocates for a sporting agenda that prizes the subjectivity of the individual, emphasizes the intrinsic processes of self-knowing and self-expression, and encourages independent initiative.

While we should support athletes' ambitions, we need to step back from thinking about sporting practices merely as places for seeking to maximize the achievement of individual athletes and teams for economic profit or political propaganda. Sport is more than performance—more than running faster, jumping higher, and throwing farther. Privileging performance enhancement in sport over other processes and outcomes that are just as important is what needs problematizing.

One real challenge for all of us working in the field of physical activity is finding ways to structure sports so that participants are able to pursue their ambitions and dreams while avoiding narrow technical and instrumentally rational thinking. In other words, the challenge is finding ways to use sport for self-expression, self-enhancement, self-esteem development, and personal social development. As Mike Messner (1987) has said, "since the sports world is an important cultural arena that serves partly to socialize [participants] to hierarchical, competitive, and aggressive values, it is also an important context within which to confront the needs for a humanizing of [people]" (pp. 65-66).

Moreover, if meanings in sports are really part of a "contested terrain," if they are part of a larger component of political, economic, and cultural conflicts, the outcomes of which are *not* naturally preordained to favor capital and the politically powerful, then the demanding and unceasing daily struggle at the level of research about sports must be part of these larger conflicts as well.

In this vein, sport scientists need to become active agents in contesting dominant social discourses by incorporating moral and political issues into sports discourses while joining those day-to-day struggles within sports to other actions promoting a more progressive society in the wider social arena. I'm reminded of the insightful comment of the late Red Smith, one of the most admired sports-

---

[2]*The New York Times* (Nov. 17, 1989) estimated that 50% of the 9,000 athletes who competed at the 1988 Seoul Olympics were using drugs. In 1989, Bill Fralic of the Atlanta Falcons, testifying before the Biden Senate Committee, said that the use of steroids was rampant in the NFL, intercollegiate athletics, and high school athletics.

writers, that any sportswriter who thinks the world is no bigger than the outfield fence is not only a bad citizen but also a lousy sportswriter. We might make a similar statement for the sport scientist who thinks sports are no bigger than performance enhancement.

Although well intentioned, the discourse of performance enhancement subordinates and marginalizes moral, ritual, experiential, and social discourses that were historically a part of sport. As Kidd (1990) has argued,

> The current regime of high performance sport . . . is particularly dehumanizing. It is not just the devaluing of athletes' intrinsic worth by the overwhelming emphasis upon medals and winners, . . . but the requirement that athletes mould their bodies and minds solely to the demands of their sports. . . . This is not the clandestine activity of a few, but the central focus of the entire sports system, not only coaches, but physiologists, biochemists, biomechanists, and [psychologists], aided by "legal" drugs and performance-enhancing practices . . . and the latest technical equipment and research. (p. 6)

I want to emphasize that critical social thought applied to sport is not critical simply in the sense of expressing disapproval of contemporary sport forms and practices; instead, its intent is to emphasize that the role of sport scientists needs to be expanded beyond understanding, predicting, and controlling to consider the ways in which the social formations of sport can be improved, made more democratic, socially just, and humane.

By making problematic the dominant discourses, values, and traditions in our everyday life, by encouraging reflective analysis of and moral deliberation over the dilemmas of sport, we can increase "the possibility of human agency in providing for a social transformation that creates new social structures and transformative conditions" (Popkewitz, 1984, p. 17).

The essential link between theory, research, and practical critical science is through political and social engagement aimed at the transformation of individual and collective practices. One obvious implication of this is that scientists must become participants in the world and thus part of the ongoing structural relations as well as being implicated in shaping debates. Unlike researchers from traditions that seek to merely understand, critical scientists aspire to transform the present and produce a different and better future (Fay, 1987). Thus they take on the role of critical observers who speak with a voice of social consciousness.

Embodied in critical social thought is an action oriented commitment to the common welfare. That we are all active agents in the construction of our social world and our personal lives is a fundamental principle. Accordingly, we "can be the subjects, rather than the objects, of socio-historical processes" (Comstock, 1982, p. 371), and we can create our own history by transforming social structures instead of being dominated by them (Flacks, 1988). Thus, a fundamental "practical interest in the fate and quality of social and political life . . . in radically improving human existence" is embraced (Bernstein, 1976, pp. 174, 180).

Concluding Remarks

In conclusion, the popularity of high performance sport will undoubtedly continue to exert strong demands for kinesiologists to assist coaches, trainers, and athletes in achieving new performance records. Yet research and professional services by academicians in the service of gathering data and providing services for sports practices, whose major purpose is helping corporations find new ways to make more money and advancing governmental interests, merits our serious thoughts and reflections.

We might hope that alternative predilections will emerge in which scholars and professionals in our field direct their efforts and energies toward examining the moral and political implications of the cult of performance enhancement in sport, studying ways in which sport participation might be evaluated by qualitative criteria rather that by abstract efficiency criteria, and viewing sports in the context of broad social issues of power and ideology (Sage, 1990).

We are all learners and teachers; as such, we can teach each other and learn from each other. Exposure to different perspectives enables us to envisage alternate realities, discover unexpected connections, and create new spaces of thought and reflection, all of which empowers us to think and act critically about our scholarly and professional work.

As long as our many voices and many perspectives are heard, and as long as we create opportunities like this to come together to speak and listen, and to articulate our distinctive perspectives, a durable and worthwhile common understanding can emerge out of our multiple intelligences. I hope my remarks contribute in some small way to advancing reflections about the problematics of performance enhancement in sport and thus broadening the discourse about meanings and ends in sport.

References

Alt, J. (1983). Sport and cultural reification: From ritual to mass consumption. *Theory, Culture, & Society*, **1**, 93-107.

Bernstein, R.J. (1976). *The restructuring of social and political theory*. New York: Harcourt Brace Jovanovich.

Bok, D. (1986). *Higher learning*. Cambridge, MA: Harvard University Press.

Bredo, E., & Feinberg, W. (1982). Conclusion: Action, interaction, self-reflection. In E. Bredo & W. Feinberg (Eds.), *Knowledge and values in social and educational research* (pp. 423-442). Philadelphia: Temple University Press.

Carr, W., & Kemmis, S. (1986). *Becoming critical: Education, knowledge and action*. Philadelphia: Falmer Press.

Coakley, J. (1989, November). *The use of performance enhancing drugs: A case of positive deviance*. Paper presented at the annual conference of the North American Society for the Sociology of Sport, Washington, DC.

Comstock, D.E. (1982). A method for critical research. In E. Bredo & W. Feinberg (Eds.), *Knowledge and values in social and educational research* (pp. 370-390). Philadelphia: Temple University Press.

Donnelly, P. (1990). *Youth involvement in high performance sport: The good, the bad, and the ugly*. Unpublished manuscript, McMaster University, Department of Physical Education, Hamilton, ON.

Fay, B. (1987). *Critical social science: Liberation and its limits*. Ithaca, NY: Cornell University Press.

Feldman, J. (1989). *Universities in the business of repression.* Boston: South End Press.

Flacks, R. (1988). *Making history: The American left and the American mind.* New York: Columbia University Press.

Foucault, M. (1977). *Discipline and punish: The birth of the prison.* New York: Pantheon.

Foucault, M. (1979). *The history of sexuality, Vol. 1: An introduction.* London: Allen Lane.

Gibson, R. (1986). *Critical theory and education.* London: Hodder and Stoughton.

Gruneau, R. (1979). Power and play in Canadian social development. *Working papers in the sociological study of sports and leisure,* **2**(1), 1-68.

Gruneau, R. (1989). Making spectacle: A case study in television sports production. In L.A. Wenner (Ed.), *Media, sports, & society* (pp. 134-154). Newbury Park, CA: Sage.

Habermas, J. (1970). *Toward a rational society.* Boston: Beacon.

Harvey, J. (1986). The rationalization of bodily practices. *Arena Review,* **10**, 55-65.

Jacoby, R. (1987). *The last intellectuals: American culture in the age of academe.* New York: Basic.

Kidd, B. (1990, September). *A new orientation to the Olympic Games.* Paper presented at After the Dubin Inquiry: Implications for Canada's High Performance Sport System conference, Queen's University, Kingston, ON.

Lynton, E.A. (1987). *New priorities for the university: Meeting society's needs for applied knowledge and competent individuals.* San Francisco: Jossey-Bass.

McKay, J., Gore, J.M., & Kirk, D. (1990). Beyond the limits of technocratic physical education. *Quest,* **42**, 52-76.

Messner, M.A. (1987). The life of a man's seasons. In M.S. Kimmel (Ed.), *Changing men: New directions in research on men and masculinity* (pp. 53-67). Newbury Park, CA: Sage.

Mills, C.W. (1959). *The sociological imagination.* New York: Oxford University Press.

Popkewitz, T.S. (1984). *Paradigm and ideology in educational research.* New York: The Falmer Press.

Popkewitz, T.S. (1989, March). *Whose future? Whose past? Notes on a critical science and methodology.* Paper presented at the Phi Delta Kappa International Alternative Paradigms Conference, San Francisco.

Sage, G.H. (1990). *Power and ideology in American sport: A critical perspective.* Champaign, IL: Human Kinetics.

Shapiro, S. (1990). *Between capitalism and democracy.* New York: Bergin & Garvey.

Turner, B.S. (1982). The discourse of diet. *Theory, Culture, & Society,* **1**, 23-32.

Weber, M. (1938). *The rules of sociological method* (8th ed.). Chicago: University of Chicago Press.

Whitson, D. (1984). Sport and hegemony: On the construction of the dominant culture. *Sociology of Sport Journal,* **1**, 64-78.

Whitson, D.J., & Macintosh, D. (1990). The scientization of physical education: Discourses of performance. *Quest,* **42**, 40-51.

Wilshire, B. (1990). *The moral collapse of the university.* Albany: State University of New York Press.

Modifying the Performance Enhancement Ethos: Disciplinary and Professional Implications

Janet C. Harris
University of North Carolina at Greensboro

Many well-known scholars are content to rest in the theoretical niches that they have carved out for themselves. Not only are they comfortable there, but others constantly situate them there and it becomes very difficult to overcome inertia and make major theoretical moves. Perhaps a sign of a truly great scholar is resistance to such tendencies marked by continued questioning of favorite frameworks and searching for better ones that offer greater insightfulness and sophistication. It is clear that Sage has continued to do this throughout his career, and I consider this to be highly commendable.

Sage's Leftist Critique:
Expansion, Review, and Extension

Where has Sage moved recently? The answer is to contemporary, leftist-based social theory stemming from Marxism! The former collegiate basketball coach, who for many years as a scholar has used humanistic arguments to critique athletics in general and intercollegiate athletics in particular, has now given his critique a Marxist coloring. Those with even cursory knowledge of the social sciences need only glance at the title of his recent undergraduate textbook, *Power and Ideology in American Sport* (1990), to realize his new orientation.

Actually the move is not as dramatic as it might at first appear. His humanistic critique has centered around the inhumane climate that intercollegiate athletics offers collegiate athletes. Rather than providing programs that help to enhance development of college students in multifaceted ways—the major goal of any university's total undergraduate program—intercollegiate athletic programs, he would argue, have in many cases served as obstructions that prevent athletes from developing their human potential to the fullest.

Old-style Marxism and the various contemporary, revised versions of it are critical of capitalistic systems on similar grounds: the failure of these systems to provide opportunities for *all* of the people to develop their human potential to the fullest. The relevant Marxist concept here is alienation stemming from the capitalistic economic system—alienation of various segments of society from one another, and alienation of people from their own full humanness and their own bodies. This alienation is thought to be rooted in the values of those who control production processes, values oriented toward considering workers to be expendable, machine-like components in the commodity system.

Remember that Marxism developed in the middle of the industrial revolution as a critique of the squalor in which the new working class was forced to live, and the generally inhumane regard for workers that many owners of industry seemed to exhibit. Unequal power relationships between workers and owners were thought to be at the crux of the problem.

More recently in leftist social thinking, the concept of power relationships has been broadened beyond socioeconomic groups such as workers and owners to include greater emphasis on power relations among males and females, racial groups, age groups, and a variety of other social constituencies. Inequality in power is thought to be at the root of lack of social justice—lack of opportunity for *all* of the people to develop their human potential to the fullest.

So Sage has not moved so far theoretically after all. He is still interested in transforming sport so that it can provide maximum opportunity for multifaceted human development, and he has found that leftist-based scholarship provides useful insights about barriers to reaching this goal, especially in terms of barriers presented by power relationships among numerous societal groups (cf. Gruneau, 1983; Whitson, 1984).

Various strains of Marxist thought are especially useful for bringing to light the role that commercialization of sport in American society has played in preventing sport from becoming a venue for maximizing human potential. Sage's presentation pointed to the importance of commercialization as a factor underlying the strength of the performance enhancement ethos.

In my opinion, his leftist-based thinking has sharpened his arguments and made them stronger and more explicit. If we take his critique of high performance, elite sport to heart, the implications for changes in our discipline and profession are quite profound and far-reaching. We would need a major overhaul of the questions we ask as scholars and the sorts of tasks that we and our students set about doing as professionals. We will return to this shortly.

Let us first recall Sage's main points. His analysis turned on *making problematic* the seemingly very natural and easily accepted assumption that our discipline and profession should be directed toward performance enhancement in sport, especially elite sport. This assumption of course underlies the main theme of this year's Academy program. How many of you, upon learning of the program topic, asked yourself whether performance enhancement in sport is something we ought to be doing in our field? If you did not, I suspect you are in good company. Your failure even to raise the question privately in your own thoughts is a good example of how ingrained and natural the value of performance enhancement in sport has become.

This ethos or world view, in his words, is rooted in a "scientized, technocratic, instrumentally rational" view of human beings, along with the assumption that our current sport forms and the governing structures in which the sport forms are embedded are in no need of criticism.

However, neither the technocratic view of human beings nor our current sport forms and governing organizations is immutable, cast in concrete for all time. These features of life in our society, along with all the rest of our social life, are socially constructed: They have evolved out of continuous social interaction, and they will change as a result of future social interaction. They do not constitute *the* natural order of things; rather they are one way of doing things. An infinite number of alternatives could be developed in their place.

It is clear that the performance enhancement ethos is central to sports that are popular in American society. Acceptance of this mentality by sport scientists of course leads to engaging in efforts to enhance performance, but beyond this it also gives tacit acknowledgment and support to our dominant sport enterprise—elite youth and scholastic sports, big-time collegiate sports, professional sports, and elite American teams that compete internationally.

If we accept Sage's notion that the current penchant in American society for performance enhancement in sport is an ethos or world view that is open to question, and if we also agree with him that our current, almost single-minded focus on performance enhancement presents serious barriers to enhancing other aspects of human functioning in and through sport, then this suggests that the current emphasis by sport scientists on ways to enhance performance needs reexamination and alteration.

Sage asked us to consider how we can encourage performance enhancement in sport and at the same time encourage maximum, multifaceted human development instead of producing narrow, one-sided athletic automatons focused single-mindedly on ever and ever greater athletic feats. He pointed out that performance enhancement is not the only goal worth pursuing for sport scientists but that we should also explore "the ways in which the social formations of sport can be improved, made more democratic, socially just, and humane."

Sage emphasized the deleterious effects on athletes of the performance enhancement ethos, saying that "the athlete's body has become an instrument, an object to be worked on, trained, tuned, and manipulated in order to achieve maximum performance." Beyond personal developmental problems for high performance athletes, however, the intense focus on performance enhancement has broader social repercussions, which Sage alluded to without going into detail.

His two questions, Performance enhancement for whom? Performance enhancement for what purposes? were tied primarily to concerns about problems faced by individual athletes vis-à-vis commercially controlled, technocratic sport. However, these questions could just as easily have led him to a more detailed exploration of limitations on social justice and equal opportunity in sport faced by various constituencies in American society, constituencies based on such factors as race, socioeconomic status, gender, age, sexual preference, ethnicity, geography, and vocational and avocational interests.

Let us explore this a little further. Commercialization has elevated particular sports to a level of importance warranting large expenditures of money to employ science and technology to enhance performance and increase the chances of winning. Spectators who pay to watch are oriented toward wanting ever better levels of performance, and the sport industry attempts to give them what they want. Commercialization has resulted in mass appeal of a small number of sports—especially football, basketball, baseball, and boxing in American society, along with a variety of Olympic sports—and marginalization of a vast array of other sports and sports performance styles that reflect the mutlicultural nature of society.

Our concerns for performance enhancement do not usually extend beyond sports that are commercially valuable. This suggests that a third question be added to Sage's other two: What sorts of performances should be enhanced?

For example, before we set about enhancing the performance of young black basketball players in inner-city ghettos, we should be certain that we understand the nature of the performance qualities and styles they value. There is anecdotal and scholarly evidence that inner-city black and suburban white basketball styles are quite different (Axthelm, 1982; Carlston, 1983; Kochman, 1981). The black style is flashy and individualistic while the white style is more deliberate and team oriented. In the case of the flamboyant, dazzling black style, it might be appropriate to provide choreographers along with sport scientists to aid in enhancing performance.

There is debate about the origins of these differences, but the point for us here is that it seems important to recognize and accommodate such differences in our quest to enhance performance. If we do not, we are likely to end up with a bland, competitive sameness that obliterates multicultural diversity. Unfortunately, commercialization of a few sports and particular playing styles and marginalization of most others seems to have already led in this direction.

Interestingly, in the case of black and white basketball styles, my own casual observations suggest that the "white game" is more acceptable at the collegiate level while the "black game" is more in vogue at the professional level. Rules preventing zone defenses at the professional level and allowing them at the collegiate level encourage these two different styles. The ways in which these different styles became articulated at the two levels of the game would be an interesting topic for further study.

It is important to note, however, that emphasis on the black playing style at one level of highly commercialized sport and the white playing style at another is evidence that not all local playing styles necessarily are obliterated by commercialization and related technologically based performance enhancement processes.

With this last point in mind, we might ask whether it is beneficial to either style to be caught up in commercialized, technocratic sport. When commercial interests control the shaping and reshaping of playing styles—the nature of the performance that is to be the focus of performance enhancement—control of the way in which the game is played moves away from players and their local constituencies and into the hands of management and their hired coaches, sport scientists, and marketing experts.

It is beyond the scope of this presentation to explore this last idea fully, but it seems rather clear that technocratic performance enhancement in the service of commercialized sport is likely to remove much of the opportunity for athletes to control the shape of their own playing styles. Going even further, it would be completely out of the question for them to start playing an entirely different sport that is of interest to their own local social constituencies.

Implications for the Discipline and the Profession

The critique of performance enhancement in sport presented by Sage and expanded somewhat here has profound implications for our discipline and profession. Sage encouraged us to be active as sport scientists in considering "the ways in which . . . sport can be improved, made more democratic, socially just, and humane."

There is a running debate in the social sciences about the desirability of scholars becoming actively involved in grass-roots social change, and some would argue that uncovering social problems through research and making those known to others is all that can be expected. I do not intend to add to this debate here, but rather to move in a different direction to examine what we might do to change our discipline and related professions to address the problems that surround the enhancement of performance in sport.

Let us first consider the discipline. Recall that Sage urged us to look beyond our current, uncritical acceptance of the worth of performance enhancement. He suggested that we ask different, critical questions: "Performance enhancement for whom? Performance enhancement for what purposes?" and I have added, What sorts of performances should be enhanced?

Several avenues of inquiry can be listed that are likely to provide us with unsettling answers to these and other questions dealing with the worth of intense, single-minded attention to performance enhancement in sport: sociocultural research on power relationships in sport and the larger society in which sport is embedded; philosophical research on ethics in sport; historical research on the rise of commercialized sport; psychological research on stress and enjoyment in sport; and biomedical research on atheletes' health and well-being.

Those in our discipline who have been asking and answering unsettling questions about sport are in the extreme minority, of course, and most are certainly not in the mainstream of the field. They work in the margins of the discipline, tolerated in most cases as vestiges of some earlier era when the bulk of scholars in our field held more eclectic views of its central missions. No matter how articulate and well supported their research, their refusal to accept sport as it is currently constituted brands them at times as pariahs.

The fact that most of the unsettling questions and answers have come from research within social science and humanities frameworks makes it especially easy for those in psychobiological areas (the majority of scholars in our field) to dismiss it. Such work can easily be pigeonholed as being beyond one's own specialized scholarly competence, and thus it can easily be ignored as not relevant to one's own academic endeavors.

Countering this, Sage suggested, and I agree, that it is important for *all* sport scientists to revisit the unexamined assumption that research geared toward enhancing performance in sport should be paramount above work oriented toward (a) critiquing the current intense focus on performance enhancement and (b) enhancing broad human development and social justice in sport. Scholars who approach sport using social science and humanities frameworks are in a good position to lead the field in this endeavor because of the critical questions they typically ask.

This leadership will lead nowhere, however, unless those doing performance enhancement research are open to serious soul-searching and possible reorientation of their work. This is not easy to do, and whether it will happen in the future is highly open to question.

Let us turn now to consider sport related professions. These include coaching, athletic training, teaching, sport management, recreation management, scholarly consulting and research for the athletic industry, and others as well. If we are concerned about the problems surrounding performance enhancement in sport, then we should, in the professional training we offer to future sport professionals, include opportunities for critical examination of the whole performance enhancement endeavor. Critical examination of performance enhancement is only one aspect of a much broader critical examination of sport that seems desirable to incorporate in the training we provide.

Not all would agree that we should be training critical professionals. After all, our field is still attempting to legitimize itself as a discipline and a profession. We are still in a somewhat tenuous position in this regard.

Lawson (1985) went so far as to suggest that we should "expect to confront the challenges of deprofessionalization" (p. 20) because we have not been able to monopolize either the generation of our own knowledge or the use of it by professionals whom we train. Furthermore, even professions with solid, longstanding legitimacy such as law or medicine must maintain relatively conservative postures in terms of socializing new recruits into their ranks in order to ensure self-preservation.

With this in mind, it may be folly to suggest that we should work to produce young critical professionals—radicals who would not necessarily be followers of our conventional wisdom. We might end up destroying our field altogether. Nevertheless, if we want to produce thoughtful professionals who are willing and able to raise questions about crucial matters such as the level of support that our field should give to performance enhancement, then such an approach may be called for.

How do we go about training critical professionals, and what would these people do differently from more conservative professionals once they are on the job? Let us first consider the latter question. The traditional view of professionals is that they possess a stock of specialized knowledge and skills valued by the public. This is usually gained through advanced academic training. Professionals provide scarce and valued services to society, and they receive money or other forms of compensation in return.

The assumption is that professionals know what people need and want, and that *they* know how best to deliver it. Once the public decides that a certain group of professionals has valuable services to offer, most of the power is in the hands of the professionals themselves in terms of deciding the specifics of rendering service.

Leaving aside difficult questions about whether or not theoretical/scientific knowledge in our field transfers readily into practical knowledge and action (Lawson, 1985, 1990), this traditional view of professionals is problematic from the standpoint of inequalities in power between the professionals and the people they serve. Traditional professionals have little interest in permitting local constituencies to advise them and help with tailoring their services to fit local needs and interests. They believe they know best what is needed.

If it is important for various constituencies in American society to have influence over the shaping of their own lives, then it is crucial that professionals attempt to adjust and alter their services to fit in with local social situations. What might critical professionals do that could help them mold their services to be in tune with the traditional social life of the people they set out to help?

Scholars studying the medical profession (Freidson, 1970) and social services fields (Galper, 1975) have addressed this concern. Three suggestions can be offered: First, critical professionals should put themselves in positions in which they interact frequently with colleagues in other related fields, with the goal of becoming more aware of local societal problems from perspectives beyond those of their own profession. Ideally this would prod them to look beyond the conventional wisdom of their own discipline and profession in forming opinions about how to proceed with providing services.

Second, local people who are the recipients of professional services should be closely involved in the overall planning of programs. Third, if choices must be made between specific local groups that will receive services, more success may be achieved in getting local people involved in the planning if groups are selected that already show some level of self-initiative, such as raising money or finding their own leaders to help further their goals.

These strategies should help critical professionals in sport settings to enhance performance in sport while at the same time attempting to ensure that (a) local sports and local playing styles are maintained, and (b) sport is shaped to provide opportunities for *everyone* to develop his or her human potential to the fullest. The sorts of questions raised earlier should help clarify the kind of guidance that critical professionals might seek from the recipients of their services: "Performance enhancement for whom? Performance enhancement for what purposes? What sorts of performances should be enhanced?"

It would be relatively easy to involve grass-roots constituencies in thinking about performance enhancement priorities and strategies at the level of marginalized, local sports that are of minor commercial interest. Players themselves as well as others in local communities could be involved in planning and implementing programs. The fact that sport scientists and sport professionals generally pay little attention to sports and playing styles at this level is perhaps a testament to their marginalized, trivial status.

In the case of commercialized sport, on the other hand, it seems much less likely that a grass-roots planning process would be tolerated. Those who control commercialized sports have too much at stake to risk the consequences of such dalliances. The most direct recipients of performance enhancement services, the athletes, are unlikely ever to have much input into the broad planning of performance enhancement priorities and strategies.

Altering the process by which decisions are made about the emphasis needed on performance enhancement and the strategies needed to achieve it would require major restructuring of commercialized sport itself, and in my opinion this is not likely to happen soon. At this level critical professionals may be faced with unpalatable choices: not becoming involved in performance enhancement in commercialized sport at all, or being content to make relatively small changes that are responsive in a limited way to the athletes they serve.

Let us turn finally to the training of critical professionals. Three suggestions from literature about medicine, education, and our own field can be offered (Freidson, 1970; McKay, Gore, & Kirk, 1990; Schon, 1987; Zeichner & Liston, 1987). First, professional trainees should be recruited from a broad range of societal constituencies to ensure sociocultural diversity. Current calls by educational leaders for enhanced multicultural representation among our students are relevant here.

Second, professional trainees should be educated by a wide range of faculty extending beyond instructors attached directly to the profession they seek to enter. The hope is that faculty outside the profession and its underlying discipline will not be committed to the conventional wisdom of the field, and therefore students will get a variety of perspectives on their future work.

Third, reflective practicums should be established to encourage professional trainees (a) to examine their profession critically with regard to ethics and social justice issues, and (b) to build bridges between theoretical/scientific knowledge learned in school and practical knowledge learned on the job.

If we follow suggestions such as these in developing our professional training curriculums, we may find that we have a pack of young rebels on our hands. We might well create an exciting group of critical professionals who would be eager to engage in grass-roots planning of priorities and strategies for performance enhancement in settings involving marginal sports and playing styles. Perhaps the boldest among them might even take on commercialized sport and attempt to alter priorities and strategies for performance enhancement in that venue.

The danger, of course, is that the young rebels might be so disenchanted with the support given to traditional performance enhancement by our own discipline and related professions that they might suggest sweeping changes that would render our field unrecognizable to traditionalists. Such changes would be extremely hard to implement of course, but if they took hold they would be quite unsettling to many. It is hard to predict whether in the long run they would be positive or negative: They might spell the demise of our field altogether, or they might be harbingers of an invigorated rebirth.

References

Axthelm, P. (1982). *The city game*. New York: Penguin.

Carlston, D.E. (1983). An environmental explanation for race differences in basketball performance. *Journal of Sport and Social Issues*, **7**(2), 30-51.

Freidson, E. (1970). *Profession of medicine: A study of the sociology of applied knowledge*. New York: Dodd, Mead.

Galper, J.H. (1975). *The politics of social services*. Englewood Cliffs, NJ: Prentice Hall.

Gruneau, R. (1983). *Class, sports, and social development*. Amherst: University of Massachusetts Press.

Kochman, T. (1981). *Black and white styles in conflict*. Chicago: University of Chicago Press.

Lawson, H.A. (1985). Knowledge for work in the physical education profession. *Sociology of Sport Journal*, **2**, 9-24.

Lawson, H.A. (1990). Beyond positivism: Research, practice, and undergraduate professional education. *Quest*, **42**, 161-183.

McKay, J., Gore, J.M., & Kirk, D. (1990). Beyond the limits of technocratic physical education. *Quest*, **42**, 52-76.

Sage, G.H. (1990). *Power and ideology in American sport: A critical perspective*. Champaign, IL: Human Kinetics.

Schon, D.A. (1987). *Educating the reflective practitioner*. San Francisco: Jossey-Bass.

Whitson, D. (1984). Sport and hegemony: On the construction of the dominant culture. *Sociology of Sport Journal*, **1**, 64-78.

Zeichner, K.M., & Liston, D.P. (1987). Teaching student teachers to reflect. *Harvard Educational Review*, **57**(1), 23-48.

What Sport Psychology Can Contribute to the Enhancement of Human Performance

Daniel M. Landers
Arizona State University

The title of this paper relates directly to some work I have been doing for the past 7 years. Since 1984, I have participated on a committee called Techniques for the Enhancement of Human Performance. The original committee, consisting of 11 members, a chair, and a study director, was formed as a special committee of the Commission on Behavioral and Social Sciences and Education of the National Research Council/National Academy of Sciences (NRC/NAS). This NRC/NAS committee was funded by a grant from the Army Research Institute.

The basic problem was that those in decision-making roles in the U.S. Army were in a quandary over the effectiveness of several performance enhancement techniques being marketed. For example, some Army generals were favorably impressed with extraordinary techniques such as mental rehearsal and parapsychology, but other generals ranged from being mildly curious to very negative. Rather than risking the wrath of an Army general, the leadership in the Army Research Institute sought the advice of people outside of the military who were familiar with the kind of "extraordinary" psychological techniques the Army wished to have evaluated.

With the exception of myself, all of the initial committee members had degrees in psychology. It just so happened that the Army was interested in learning more about sport psychology techniques which were being promoted to enhance sport performance.

Other committee members conducted an extensive investigation into the efficacy of parapsychological techniques (i.e., remote viewing, random number generators, and Ganzfeld psi experiments) and psychological techniques, consisting of such things as sleep learning, stress management, and neurolinguistic programming. As a result of several site visits, commissioned papers, and literature reviews of both classified and unclassified scientific and anecdotal literature, the findings of the committee were published in a book (Druckman & Swets, 1988).

Within the military, the committee's report was well received, judging from their desire to extend the life of this ad hoc committee for another 2 years. The committee's charge was much the same, except that any technique having the potential of enhancing human performance, whether extraordinary or not, was to be included.

The new topics that were examined required a reorganization of the committee, with some members stepping down and five new members being added. Robert Christina joined the committee and worked with committee chair Robert Bjork on the topic of long-term retention of skills, while I reviewed literature on sport psychology techniques to optimize the preparation to perform under pressure.

Other committee members reviewed literature in the following areas that were of interest to the Army: career development, modeling experts, subliminal methods, meditation and pain management, hiding and detecting deception, and methods of enhancing group processes (e.g., decision making) to enhance human performance. The results and recommendations of the committee will soon be published (Bjork & Druckman, in press).

What I intend to present here is a summary of some of the material contained in the two papers that were most directly related to sport psychology (Landers, 1988; 1991). In the interest of economy, only the areas deemed to have a preponderance of research evidence to support an enhancement of sport or motor performance will be summarized here: (a) mental practice and motor performance, (b) cognitive-behavioral techniques and sport performance, (c) preperformance routines and sport performance, and (d) biofeedback and exercise/sport performance.

The original sources (Landers, 1988; 1991) can be consulted for a more detailed discussion and references for the areas reviewed, and for a review of the areas that were deemed as not contributing to the enhancement of sport performance (i.e., visual training programs, attentional control training, and the "static" mental health model, "iceberg profile").

Mental Practice/Motor Performance

The literature on mental practice and motor performance consists of studies conducted in a laboratory setting in which novel tasks are used to minimize the effect of prior experience and prevent practice on the task during the intervention period. Although the generalizability of these studies to sport could certainly be questioned, these studies usually contain a greater degree of experimental control (e.g., random assignment to treatment conditions, ability to maximize treatment differences among conditions) than studies conducted in a sport setting.

There have been several narrative reviews of this literature (Richardson, 1967; Singer, 1972; Weinberg, 1982) and, more recently, meta-analytic reviews have also been conducted (Feltz & Landers, 1983; Feltz, Landers, & Becker, 1988). Although the reviews have reached similar conclusions, I will focus on the results of the meta-analytic reviews since they allow a much more precise quantification of the magnitude of the performance effects produced by mental practice.

Like anything else, meta-analysis can be done poorly and thus yield biased results. However, compared to narrative reviews, with a properly conducted meta-analysis there is generally less chance for bias (Beamon, 1991): (a) it is an objective and public process; (b) all steps are included so it can be replicated; (c) it follows the rules of the scientific method; (d) it uses a metric effect size that is not influenced by sample size; and (e) by combining similarly derived effect sizes across studies, statistical power can be maximized.

In the first meta-analysis on this topic (Feltz & Landers, 1983), the effect size was calculated by subtracting the mean of the control group from the mean of the treatment group (mental practice) and dividing by the pooled standard deviation. In the second meta-analysis (Feltz et al., 1988), a learning score effect size was calculated by subtracting the mean for the posttest from the mean of the pretest and then dividing by the standard deviation for the pretest.

The advantage of converting the means and standard deviations to a common metric is that the effect size can then represent the meaningfulness of a mean difference. If the resultant effect size is less than 0.40, the meaningfulness of the difference is considered to be low. If the effect size is between 0.41 and 0.70, the difference is in the moderate range; and if the effect size is greater than 0.71, it is generally considered to be large and thus represents a very meaningful difference.

Regardless of whether group differences at the posttest (ES = 0.48 for 60 studies; Feltz & Landers, 1983) or pre/post change scores (ES = 0.47 for 55 studies; Feltz et al., 1988) were examined, the results showed that across many types of motor tasks the mental practice groups performed significantly better than control groups.

When tasks were subcategorized into tasks that primarily involved cognitive elements associated with movement, or primarily necessitated strength or motor skill, the largest effect sizes were found for motor tasks that involved a large cognitive component. For these cognitive tasks, very large effect sizes were found (>1.00), with fewer numbers of trials or practice sessions than needed to produce moderate to large effects for motor or strength tasks (Feltz & Landers, 1983).

A more interesting question that has been addressed in this literature is whether mental practice can be as good as or better than physical practice. To examine this, subjects in the mental and physical practice groups receive the same number of practice trials. In some studies, a combined-practice group receiving a 50:50 ratio of physical to mental practice trials is also included. When the pre/post change score effect sizes were examined for the various practice groups (Feltz et al., 1988), the pattern of findings across studies clearly showed that physical practice (ES = 0.79) produced more meaningful mean differences than combined (ES = 0.62), mental (ES = 0.47), and control (ES = 0.22) practice conditions.

These meta-analytic results suggested two hypotheses that could be tested in a single experimental study: (a) as the proportion of physical practice increases relative to mental or no practice, performance improves; and (b) compared to a motor task, tasks with more cognitive components have larger effects, even with a lesser amount of practice.

To test these hypotheses, Hird, Landers, Thomas, and Horan (1991) compared different ratios of physical to mental practice on cognitive task (pegboard) performance, which requires perceptual and symbolic task elements, and motor task (pursuit rotor) performance. Subjects (36 males and 36 females) were randomly assigned to one of the following six groups: motivational control (practice on a stabilometer), physical practice, mental practice, or one of three combined physical/mental practice groups (i.e., 75:25, 50:50, and 25:75).

There were seven practice sessions, consisting of four trials/session for the pegboard and eight trials/session for the pursuit rotor. All groups except the control group for the pegboard task improved from pretest to posttest. Consistent with the Feltz and Landers (1983) meta-analysis, effect-size calculations indicated that mental practice was more effective for the pegboard than for the pursuit rotor. The linear trend analyses and effect sizes for the posttest scores of both tasks showed that as the relative proporation of physical practice increased, performance was enhanced.

The meta-analytic findings and the Hird et al. (1991) findings indicate that for novel tasks like these, reducing or replacing physical practice with mental practice would be counterproductive if performance enhancement were the only consideration. However, for conditions wherein physical practice may be expensive, time-consuming, fatiguing, or injurious, combined mental and physical practice or mental practice alone is clearly more effective than no practice at all.

Cognitive-Behavioral Interventions and Sport Performance

The motor performance findings may not generalize to competitive sport since in sport mental practice is more likely to be used as a supplement to physical training rather than replacement for all or some of it. Because of the limited number of sport studies that have used real athletes performing in a noncontrived competitive situation in the sport in which they regularly competed, the scope of existing reviews has been broadened to include a number of mental strategies that "emphasize cognitions, thoughts, or mental activities as mediational processes and/or as central change mechanisms" (Whelan, Meyers, & Berman, 1989).

Collectively these strategies have been called "cognitive-behavioral interventions," which have consisted of imagery, relaxation, biofeedback, hypnotherapy, cognitive restructuring, systematic desensitization, self-monitoring, performance-contingent rewards, and goal setting.

A narrative review of cognitive-behavioral interventions on sport performance (Greenspan & Feltz, 1989) contained 19 published articles (23 interventions), and a meta-analytic review of this literature (Whelan et al., 1989) dealt with 49 published articles (121 comparisons across 333 outcome measures).

The overall results of these reviews provided strong support for a relationship between cognitive-behavioral interventions and an enhancement of sport performance. For instance, Whelan et al. (1989) found that the average effect size represented over half a standard deviation advantage (ES = 0.62) in the performance of athletes receiving cognitive-behavioral interventions compared to control groups who were denied this supplemental training. Likewise, Greenspan and Feltz (1989) observed the same facilitation of sport performance in 87% of the studies in their review.

It is unlikely that these results are spurious due to not including unpublished master's theses or doctoral dissertations, since application of Orwin's (1983) fail-safe formula shows that it would take at least 120 unpublished studies having an effect size of 0.20 or less to reduce Whelan et al.'s 0.62 effect size to an effect size of 0.20.

A closer examination of these and other reviews suggests some of the moderating factors that may be important in producing better sport performance. For instance, relative to athletes not receiving cognitive-behavioral interventions, athletes who received them performed better when (a) there was an objective out-come measure of performance; (b) the intervention contained multiple compo-nents (e.g., relaxation + imagery + biofeedback); (c) they employed many training sessions in the intervention presented to the atheletes and conducted these sessions live as opposed to an audiotape; (d) they were involved in sports in which there was direct competition with others; and (e) they were performing sport skills containing a high degree of perceptual or symbolic elements (i.e., relatively more cognitive) or sport skills involving accuracy, endurance, and strength (with more sessions or trials than for cognitive-motor tasks).

Although few studies have used cognitive-behavioral interventions with elite athletes at the Olympic or professional level, three of the four studies using elite performers (see Greenspan & Feltz, 1989) showed positive effects of cognitive-behavioral interventions on sport performance.

The most convincing evidence, which was derived from a study employing a true experimental design, is the study by Kim (1989). In this study, Olympic rifle shooters were randomly assigned in equal numbers ($n=12$) to four groups: a relaxation/imagery group, a meditation/imagery group, a combined relaxa-tion/imagery/meditation group, and a no-treatment control group. The subjects in the first three groups listened to audiotapes in a private room two times a day over a 6-week period (total = 13 hrs), while subjects in the control group listened to classical music for the same amount of time.

Kim (1989) found no pretest differences among groups, but there were significant pretest/posttest differences for anxiety and performance. Although no differences were found for relaxation/imagery and control groups, the medita-tion/imagery and the combined meditation/relaxation/imagery groups showed significant posttest reductions in self-reported anxiety and better shooting performance.

Analysis of posttest scores only revealed a signficant difference among groups for shooting performance ($p<.05$), and Scheffé post hoc tests showed that this was due to the combined group performing better than the control group. Secondary analysis of Kim's (1989, Table 1) data revealed that the relaxation/medi-tation/imagery training group was more effective in reducing anxiety (ES = 0.93) and improving performance (ES = 0.80) than the meditation/imagery (ES = 0.48 and 0.24, respectively), relaxation/imagery (ES = 0.30 and -0.14, respectively), and control (ES = -0.04 and 0.04, respectively) groups. Kim's findings sup-port other investigators' (Smith, 1980; Suinn, 1983) contention that the effects of interventions used with elite athletes may be more beneficial if multicompo-nent treatments are employed.

Although the research evidence in the motor performance and sport literature generally supports the effectiveness of imagery and other cognitive-behavioral techniques in improving sport performance, some sport psychologists are con-cerned that the techniques taught to athletes in noncompetitive settings may not generalize to performance when under intense competitive pressure. The basic premise of this type of research is that the few seconds preceding the execution of a motor or sport skill are critical for successful performance.

Whether athletes have good mental control the day before or an hour before competition may have litle to do with the control they exhibit immediately prior to performance. By training athletes to incorporate cognitive-behavioral techniques into a preperformance routine, or ritual, it is believed that athletes' levels of concentration will be enhanced and thus their performance will be better or more consistent.

Preperformance Routines and Sport Performance

Structured preperformance routines have typically been used by experienced performers executing skill activities wherein the environment is static (e.g., tennis serve, golf putt, archery, riflery). According to Crews and Boutcher (1986), the preperformance routine consists of "a set pattern of cue thoughts, actions, and images consistently carried out before performance of the skill" (p. 291).

Crews and Boutcher maintain that athletes have learned the preperformance routine "to divert attention away from negative, irrelevant information, to stop attention focusing on a well-learned skill [e.g., disruption of automatic processing], and to establish the appropriate physical and mental state for the ensuing task" (p. 291). In practice, it is assumed that if athletes do not have a well-established preperformance routine, they should develop one by drawing from the cognitive-behavioral techniques in which they are already proficient.

There are commercially available preperformance routines, for example Loehr's mental toughness training program (1989) (see Table 1). There is also an emerging sport science literature on preperformance routines. For example, Crews and Boutcher (1986) assigned 15 golfers from a beginning golf class to an experimental, preshot routine group (i.e., employing cognitive-behavioral skills described in the previous section) and 15 to a control (no preshot routine) group.

Following an 8-week preshot routine training program, Crews and Boutcher (1986) found that the performance of the preshot routine group improved, but only for the more proficient male golfers. It was concluded that preshot routine training improved performance when physical skills were well learned. In another study of 12 collegiate golfers (Boutcher & Crews, 1987), both males and females improved the consistency of the preshot routine behaviors following a 6-week training period, but only the females improved in task performance.

Preshot routines have also been effective in improving basketball free-throw shooting performance (Lobmeyer & Wasserman, 1986) and novel motor task performance (Singer, Flora, & Abpirezl, 1989). Following a preshot training program, subjects made a 7% improvement in performance when using their preshot routine compared to when they were not using the routine (Lobmeyer & Wasserman, 1986). In a laboratory environment, subjects ($n=10$) were taught a five-step learning strategy that sequentially consisted of "Readying → Imaging → Focusing → Executing → Evaluating" (Singer et al., 1989). Following four practice trials, subjects in the learning strategy group performed significantly faster, but not at the expense of more errors, than the control group and the group that previewed the location of the six targets.

In summary, in most studies, subjects reported that a preperformance routine increased their concentration. In addition, in the majority of the studies the preperformance routine led to better performance (i.e., in five out of eight comparisons the gains were statistically significant).

Interview data from athletes and the general assumptions of investigators support the idea that a preperformance routine increases the performer's concentration

Table 1

Loehr's Mental Toughness Training Program

Response stages	Time following last point	Example behaviors
Positive physical response	3–5 s	Clap for opponents, clench fists, walk briskly back to baseline
Relaxation response	6–15 s	Walk back and forth until breathing and heart rate stabilize; relax arms and hands, stretch, take deep breaths
Preparation response	16–21 s	Move toward baseline and direct lift of eyes to opposite court, strong statement with momentary pause to review score and intentions
Ritual response	22–30 s	Step to baseline, adjust arousal levels and deepen concentration; bounce ball and pause after last bounce; stimulate feet; only think about serve and not technical aspects of tennis

and facilitates performance. Although athletes who are given training in a preperformance routine report better concentration, retrospective reports of cognitive processes are known to be unreliable (Nisbett & Wilson, 1977).

Likewise, trying to obtain self-reports during the preperformance routine is counterproductive since it will interfere with the desired state of automatic processing in the moments before response execution. However, there are electrophysiological indicators of attention that have been used with athletes who are executing their preperformance routines immediately prior to performance of a discrete, closed skill that involves minimal movement.

These studies (Landers et al., 1991; Salazar et al., 1990) basically show that (a) the preperformance routines of elite and pre-elite archers are associated with electrophysiological changes (i.e., heart rate deceleration and EEG hemispheric asymmetry) that affect performance; and (b) disruption of archers' normal preperformance mental routine (e.g., by learning an incorrect EEG pattern through biofeedback training) will result in significantly poorer performance. Using biofeedback in this way is unique and therefore deserves greater elaboration as one of many cognitive-behavioral techniques that have the potential, if used correctly, to enhance sport performance.

Biofeedback and Sport Performance

Biofeedback, the provision of information regarding one's own biological functioning, has as its main goal the development of self-regulation. It consists of feeding physiological information back to the subject's auditory or visual senses after this information has been amplified by polygraphs, computers, and other physiological equipment. Through such training, the goal is to get the individual to regulate desired changes without instrumentation.

A number of reviews on biofeedback and sport performance have appeared in the literature (Landers, 1988; Lawrence, 1984; Lawrence & Johnson, 1977; Zaichowsky & Fuchs, 1988). Taken together, these reviews have concluded that performance improvements (a) have not been consistently demonstrated with either EMG or alpha enhancement biofeedback, and (b) have been shown for heart rate biofeedback and slow potential biofeedback.

Other types of biofeedback have been examined with respect to motor performance (e.g., thermal, multiple autonomic responses, event related potentials), but these have not been shown to be directly relevant for sport and exercise and therefore will not be discussed (see Landers, 1988, for reviews of these areas).

Heart Rate Biofeedback

Since the mid-1970s, research has examined the efficacy of biofeedback in the regulation of heart rate (HR) response to exercise. Many of these studies have examined the clinical benefits for middle-age hypertensive and cardiac patients, but enough research has been conducted with healthy subjects to suggest that aerobic physical capacities could possibly be enhanced through biofeedback.

In terms of HR attenuation during dynamic exercise, Engel's work has been at the forefront. Engel and his colleagues have been able to demonstrate with both medical (Fredrikson & Engel, 1985) and normal adult populations (Perski & Engel, 1980; Perski, Tzankoff, & Engel, 1985) that subjects receiving HR feedback to help them lower their heart rate had an exercise HR that was 20–22% lower than that of control subjects who exercised with no feeback.

Of greater relevance to sport performance is the application of Engel's research to well-conditioned subjects (VO_2max $\geq$ 45 ml/kg/min) performing at higher exercise intensities (e.g., 65% of HR max). Perski et al. (1985) randomly assigned 10 physically fit males to either a nonfeedback control group or a HR feedback group. All subjects exercised for approximately 21 min/day over 4 consecutive days. Subjects performed five 4.25-min workloads at 65% of HR max, as determined from a maximal exercise test, with a 2-min rest period separating each workload. While they were cycling, feedback subjects could choose which of three visual HR feedback displays they would use to reduce HR.

The results indicated that subjects given HR feedback had average heart rates that were 22% less than for control subjects. The subjects also had reduced ventilation and tended to use less oxygen. These findings prompted Perski et al. (1985) to suggest that cardiovascular adjustments through biofeedback training did not change performance in the working muscles. This was further supported by the fact that blood lactate concentrations did not change. They concluded that the tendency for lower oxygen consumption after training reflected the decreased respiratory muscle demands associated with the lower ventilation.

It seems that there are positive effects from HR attenuation during dynamic exercise with intensities less than 65% of maximum, apparently without compensatory effects elsewhere. However, for these biofeedback effects to have more direct application to sport performance, the following remains to be determined: (a) whether HR attenuation can be achieved at even greater exercise intensities (e.g., >70% max); (b) whether the ability to reduce HR during exercise allows subjects to exercise for longer periods of time; and (c) whether biofeedback produces more HR attenuation than some other cognitive-behavioral technique (e.g., relaxation, imagery).

Slow Potentials

Electrical potentials of the brain that are time-locked to some evoking stimulus or event are called event related potentials. A special case of event related potentials, referred to as slow potentials, describes the slow negative potential shift that develops during a period prior to an alerting stimulus (e.g., the foreperiod in a reaction time [RT] paradigm). Such a potential occurs when two stimuli are related so that one stimulus, for example a warning stimulus, signals the presentation of an upcoming motor or mental task.

Slow potentials can be either positive or negative. Positive slow potentials are thought to reflect a consumption of cerebral resources while a negative potential, also called the contingent negative variation, is believed to be a state of preparation or mobilization of cerebral resources for the ensuing response (Birbaumer, Lutzenberger, Elbert, Rockstroh, & Schwarz, 1981).

When examined with respect to performance, research has shown that slow potentials are associated with (a) faster, less variable RT performance, (b) faster choice RT, and (c) better performance on stimulus-response pairs (Landers, 1988). Since negative slow potential shifts have been shown to be related to performance, biofeedback training to induce such shifts may also produce better performance. Lutzenberger and his colleagues (Lutzenberger, Elbert, Rockstroh, & Birbaumer, 1979, 1982; Rockstroh, Elbert, Lutzenberger, & Birbaumer, 1982) have shown that subjects trained to increase negative shifts (a) have faster RT (by 13 ms), (b) check solutions to math problems faster (by 6 s), and (c) show less performance decrements on vigilance tasks involving signal detection.

Comparison of self-reports, muscle tension, and autonomic responses revealed that those subjects who used cognitive strategies (e.g., imagery, concentration) instead of somatovisceral strategies (e.g., changes in muscle tension) were more successful in achieving the training goals (i.e., increased negativity). This relationship between slow potentials and performance has been demonstrated often enough to "promote reasonable confidence in its validity" (Landers, 1988, p. 88).

A related line of research in a sport environment has examined EEG patterns in shooters, archers, and golfers during the preparatory period prior to response execution (Crews, 1989; Hatfield, Landers, & Ray, 1984, 1987; Salazar et al., 1990). A fairly consistent finding across these studies has been that left hemisphere EEG patterns are related to performance. In the one study in which it was examined, Crews (1989) found that slow potential shifts were also related to golf putting performance.

Given the relationships between EEG spectral densities and slow potentials, we undertook a study designed to determine whether left hemisphere activity could be augmented through biofeedback procedures and whether this training would result in better archery performance (Landers et al., 1991). Following a performance pretest (27 shots at a standard archery target 45 m away), pre-elite archers ($N=24$) were randomly assigned to either (a) a correct feedback group (i.e., greater left hemisphere, low frequency activity), (b) an incorrect feedback group (i.e., greater right hemisphere, low frequency activity), or (c) a no-feedback control group. Following the treatment, subjects were posttested using the pretest protocol.

The slow potential feedback used in this study was derived from procedures described by Elbert, Rockstroh, Lutzenberger, and Birbaumer (1980). The feedback display consisted of two horizontal bar graphs, one each for the left and right hemispheres. The position of the bar was determined by the magnitude of the slow potential shift produced during the 6 s feedback trial.

The subject's goal was to move the bar (top bar for incorrect feedback group, bottom bar for correct feedback group) as far to the right side of the computer monitor as possible. Achieving this required an increased shift in either the left hemisphere (correct feedback) or the right hemisphere (incorrect feedback). An initial criterion of a $-16\ _\mu$V slow potential shift was adjusted $\pm 2\ _\mu$V after every 6 s feedback trial, depending on whether the subject reached the criterion during the trial.

The results indicated that, compared to pretest scores, (a) the control group's performance did not change, (b) the group given left hemisphere feedback had significantly better performance after training, and (c) the group given right hemisphere feedback had significantly worse performance after training. Unlike the control and correct feedback groups, the incorrect feedback group had large increases in right hemisphere beta (i.e., 13–30 Hz) activity. This EEG pattern was uncharacteristic of elite archery performance (Salazar et al., 1990).

Landers et al. (1991) interpreted this increase as probably promoting cognitive processing that would essentially degrade performance. Such cognitive processing during performance is more characteristic of novice performers. It was concluded from this study that EEG biofeedback could affect performance, the direction of the effect being determined by whether the feedback was related to correct or incorrect EEG-performance correlates.

In conclusion, from the studies described above it is clear that biofeedback can affect exercise and sport performance. Unlike much of the biofeedback literature, these studies have isolated the effect of biofeedback (i.e., biofeedback was not part of a larger intervention package) and based the training criteria (i.e., HR or EEG feedback) on levels known to be correlated with effective task performance (Landers, 1988). In biofeedback research, where there is presently no knowledge of optimal levels of activity (e.g., EMG and alpha EEG), more basic research should be done to delineate activity levels associated with optimal performance in various exercise and sport activities.

References

Beamon, A.L. (1991). An empirical comparison of meta-analytic and traditional reviews. *Personality and Social Psychology Bulletin*, **17**, 252-257.

Birbaumer, N., Lutzenberger, W., Elbert, T., Rockstroh, B., & Schwarz, J. (1981). EEG and slow cortical potentials in anticipation of mental tasks with different hemispheric involvement. *Biological Psychology*, **13**, 251-260.

Bjork, R., & Druckman, D. (Eds.) (1991). *In the mind's eye: Understanding human performance*. Washington, DC: National Academy Press.

Boutcher, S.H., & Crews, D.J. (1987). The effect of a preshot attentional routine on a well-learned skill. *International Journal of Sport Psychology*, **18**, 30-39.

Crews, D.J. (1989). *The influence of attentive states on golf putting as indicated by cardiac and electrocortical activity*. Unpublished doctoral dissertation, Arizona State University.

Crews, D.J., & Boutcher, S.H. (1986). Effects of structured preshot behaviors on beginning golf performance. *Perceptual and Motor Skills*, **62**, 291-294.

Druckman, D., & Swets, J.A. (Eds.) (1988). *Enhancing human performance: Issues, theories, and techniques*. Washington, DC: National Academy Press.

Elbert, T., Rockstroh, B., Lutzenberger, W., & Birbaumer, N. (1980). Biofeedback of slow cortical potentials. I. *EEG and Clinical Neurophysiology*, **48**, 293-301.

Feltz, D.L., & Landers, D.M. (1983). The effects of mental practice on motor skill learning and performance: A meta-analysis. *Journal of Sport Psychology*, **5**, 25-57.

Feltz, D.L., Landers, D.M., & Becker, B.J. (1988). A revised meta-analysis of the mental practice literature on motor skill learning. In D. Druckman & J. Swets (Eds.), *Enhancing human performance: Issues, theories and techniques. Background papers* (pp. 1-65). Washington, DC: National Academy Press.

Fredrikson, M., & Engel, B.T. (1985). Learned control of heart rate during exercise in patients with borderline hypertension. *European Journal of Applied Physiology*, **54**, 315-320.

Greenspan, M.J., & Feltz, D.L. (1989). Psychological interventions with athletes in competitive situations: A review. *The Sport Psychologist*, **3**, 219-236.

Hatfield, B.D., Landers, D.L., & Ray, W.J. (1984). Cognitive processes during self-paced motor performance: An electroencephalographic profile of skilled marksmen. *Journal of Sport Psychology*, **6**, 42-59.

Hatfield, B.D., Landers, D.L., & Ray, W.J. (1987). Cardiovascular-CNS interactions during a self-paced, intentional attentive state: Elite marksmanship performance. *Psychophysiology*, **24**, 542-549.

Hird, J.S., Landers, D.M., Thomas, J.R., & Horan, J.J. (1991). Physical practice is superior to mental practice in enhancing cognitive and motor task performance. *Journal of Sport and Exercise Psychology*, **13**, 279-291.

Kim, G.B. (1989). Relative effectiveness of anxiety reduction techniques on levels of competitive anxiety and shooting performance. *Commemorative volume dedicated to Professor Hong-Dae Kim, Young-Nam University* (pp. 61-74). Dae-Ku, Republic of Korea: Honk-ik Publ. Co.

Landers, D.M. (1988). Improving motor skills. In D. Druckman & J.A. Swets (Eds.), *Enhancing human performance: Issues, theories, and techniques* (pp. 61-101). Washington, DC: National Academy Press.

Landers, D.M. (1991). Optimizing individual performance (pp. 193-246). In R. Bjork & D. Druckman (Eds.), *In the mind's eye: Understanding human performance.* Washington, DC: National Academy Press.

Landers, D.M., Petruzzello, S.J., Salazar, W., Crews, D.J., Kubitz, K.A., Gannon, T.L., & Han, M.W. (1991). The influence of electrocortical biofeedback on performance in pre-elite archers. *Medicine and Science in Sports and Exercise*, **23**, 123-129.

Lawrence, G.H. (1984). *Biofeedback and performance: An update* (Tech. Rep. 658). Alexandria, VA: U.S. Army Research Institute for the Behavioral and Social Sciences.

Lawrence, G.H., & Johnson, L.C. (1977). Biofeedback and performance. In J. Beatty & G. Schwartz (Eds.), *Biofeedback: Theory and research* (pp. 163-179). New York: Academic Press.

Lobmeyer, D.L., & Wasserman, E.A. (1986). Preliminaries to free throw shooting: Superstitious behavior? *Journal of Sport Behavior*, **9**, 70-78.

Loehr, J. (1989). *Mental toughness.* (Videotape available from Grand Slam Communications, 5150 Linton Blvd., Suite 420, Delray Beach, FL 33484).

Lutzenberger, W., Elbert, T., Rockstroh, B., & Birbaumer, N. (1979). The effects of self-regulation of slow cortical potentials on performance in a signal detection task. *International Journal of Neuroscience*, **9**, 175-183.

Lutzenberger, W., Elbert, T., Rockstroh, B., & Birbaumer, N. (1982). Biofeedback of slow cortical potentials and its effect on the performance in mental arithmetic tasks. *Biological Psychology*, **14**, 99-111.

Nisbett, R.E., & Wilson, T.D. (1977). Telling more than we can know: Verbal reports on mental processes. *Psychological Review*, **84**, 231-259.

Orwin, R.G. (1983). A fail-safe *N* for effect size. *Journal of Educational Statistics*, **8**, 157-159.

Perski, A., & Engel, B.T. (1980). The role of behavioral conditioning in the cardiovascular adjustment to exercise. *Biofeedback and Self-Regulation*, **5**, 91-103.

Perski, A., Tzankoff, S.P., & Engel, B.T. (1985). Central control of cardiovascular adjustments to exercise. *Journal of Applied Physiology*, **58**, 431-435.

Richardson, A. (1967). Mental practice: A review and discussion. Part 1. *Research Quarterly*, **38**, 95-107.

Rochstroh, B., Elbert, T., Lutzenberger, W., & Birbaumer, N. (1982). The effect of slow cortical potentials on response speed. *Psychophysiology*, **19**, 211-217.

Salazar, W., Landers, D.M., Petruzzello, S.J., Crews, D.J., Kubitz, K.A., & Han, M.W. (1990). Hemispheric asymmetry, cardiac response, and performance in elite archers. *Research Quarterly for Exercise and Sport*, **61**, 351-359.

Singer, R.S. (1972). *The psychomotor domain: Movement behavior.* Philadelphia: Lea & Febiger.

Singer, R.S., Flora, L.A., & Abpirezl, T.L. (1989). The effect of a five-step cognitive learning strategy on the acquisition of a complex motor task. *Journal of Applied Sport Psychology*, **1**, 98-108.

Smith, R.E. (1980). A cognitive-affective approach to stress management training for athletes. In C.H. Nadeau, W.R. Halliwell, K.M. Newell, & G.C. Roberts (Eds.), *Psychology of motor behavior and sport–1979* (pp. 54-72). Champaign, IL: Human Kinetics.

Suinn, R.M. (1983). Imagery and sports. In A.A. Sheikh (Ed.), *Imagery: Current theory, research, and application* (pp. 507-534). New York: Wiley.

Weinberg, R.S. (1981). The relationship between mental preparation strategies and motor performance: A review and critique. *Quest, 33,* 195-213.

Whelan, J.P., Meyers, A.W., & Berman, J.S. (1989, August). *Cognitive-behavioral interventions for athletic performance enhancement.* Paper presented at the annual meeting of the American Psychological Association, New Orleans.

Zaichowsky, L.D., & Fuchs, C.Z. (1988). Biofeedback applications in exercise and athletic performance. *Exercise and Sport Sciences Reviews, 16,* 381-421.

Social Psychological Contributions to Performance Enhancement

Diane L. Gill
University of North Carolina at Greensboro

My reaction to Dan Landers' paper will be general rather than based on specific points. I did not have the complete paper before writing this reaction, and thus I didn't write specific reactions. I did have a general idea of what Dan would cover, and had read through a paper (Landers, in press) reviewing similar material and reaching similar conclusions. Dan did his usual thorough review of the research in the areas that he covered, and I have no details to add to those topics. Instead, I will focus my remarks to highlight some other things that *might* have been said.

My perspective on sport and exercise psychology is different from Dan's, and I'll present a slightly different view of sport and exercise psychology's contribution to performance enhancement. Actually my general perspective could be described as between those of Dan and George Sage (see Sage's paper in this volume), so that may help put my comments into context.

Before elaborating on my general views, I will comment on some specific points raised by Dan's presentation. First, Dan, like some others who have discussed performance enhancement, lamented the lack of research with *elite* athletes. I do not lament it at all, and in fact I don't think the research lacks attention to elite athletes at all. From my view, nearly all of the sport psychology research on performance enhancement and applied sport psychology focuses on elite athletes. The so-called lack of elite athletes in the research is a sampling issue and not a question of research focus.

As I read the literature, most of the research questions are questions about elite athletes, and the aim of the research is to develop applications to enhance the performance of elite athletes. If the research is not about elite athletes, who is it about? Is it focused on "nonelite" athletes? Nonelite is a vague term that seems to include such diverse possibilities that any work directed at "nonelite" athletes is not really directed at anyone. I believe researchers ask questions about elite athletes but may not be able to get elite athletes as subjects, so they "sample" from the nearest population. If we define elite as the very top, sampling becomes impossible anyway.

We may also have a definitional problem. Intercollegiate athletes are elite from my perspective; even high school athletes are elite from my perspective. In any case, I do not see sport psychology work directed at enhancing performance for cardiac rehabilitation participants, women in recreational softball, or overweight youngsters in physical education classes. When those people are studied in sport and exercise psychology research, it is usually to "help" them move closer to the standards of elite athletes, as though the same standards apply to everyone.

Second, Dan, like some others in our field, suggested meta-analysis as a way to advance our work. Meta-analysis has some advantages over traditional reviews, and certainly it has a role in our work. But meta-analysis also has limits and raises some concerns. It is not appropriate for every potential topic, and over-emphasizing its use (e.g., suggesting that research in an area should start with meta-analysis) may deter us from more innovative topics and approaches as well as from topics that do not yield quantitative data or comparisons.

Even when meta-analysis is appropriate, it has drawbacks. First, I believe our research is narrowly focused, and meta-analysis seems to exaggerate this narrowing. Meta-analysis only works when you have several studies to put together. Moreover, meta-analysis seems to work best when all studies are essentially the same, with the same manipulations or easily classified conditions and groups, and with the same methods, measures, and analyses. Thus it is used on areas that have several studies (and we have only a few areas that have a body of similar research studies, as Dan noted). Perhaps social support or attentional training could enhance performance, but we do not have the studies to put into a meta-analysis to check.

My impression—and I acknowledge some bias—is that meta-analysis tends to focus on the information that's there. It summarizes information into main findings and eliminates extraneous or unique findings. It seems to strip away alternatives and possibilities that do not fit with the main comparison. New directions and questions may emerge from meta-analyses (the Feltz and Landers 1983 meta-analysis of mental practice is a good example of a meta-analysis that yielded research questions), but the typical questions are refinements of the main question that serve to narrow rather than broaden our inquiry.

Clear meta-analysis results emerge when the studies that go into the meta-analysis yield strong effects. Large effects may be obtained when studies have good internal validity. Often, though, good internal validity is achieved at a cost to external validity. Effects may be strengthened by eliminating extraneous variables, by using extreme levels or exaggerated manipulations, and by using homogenous samples in a controlled setting. Extraneous variables operate in the real world, conditions and manipulations are seldom as clear-cut as in the lab, and sociohistorical context has a tremendous influence on real-world sport and exercise behaviors.

Also, and this is definitely my bias, I'm uncomfortable with the sense of precision and objectivity implied with meta-analysis, and I miss the subjective interpretation of the reviewer that is eliminated in meta-analysis. Advocates of meta-analysis often imply, and somtimes state explicitly, that meta-analyses are more correct than interpretive reviews because meta-analytic reviews are quantitative and based on numbers.

A good reviewer brings knowledge of the subject (as well as other knowledge and experience) to draw insights and suggest possibilities that are not apparent in the original sources. An effect size is not an interpretation. Interpretation and insight may be subjective, but this subjective or creative side of reviews and research seems to provide the real value. Logic and numbers by themselves don't seem to be enough (although personally I like numbers and logic).

I'm glad Dan gave the major presentation; he gave a much more thorough review of sport psychology's contribution to performance enhancement than I could have. I don't do performance enhancement research as Dan discussed it, I'm not interested in doing it, and I'm not comfortable with the emphasis that performance enhancement receives within sport and exercise psychology. Actually, it is not performance enhancement per se but the limited or narrow view of performance enhancement that I'm not comfortable with, and that's what I want to discuss now.

First, we put the emphasis on performance when we should put the emphasis on the *performer*. We never question our assumptions about what enhanced performance means. We simply accept prevailing conventions and, moreover, assume that the same performance standards apply to everyone. Citius, altius, fortius—we assume everyone wants to be faster, higher, and stronger (perhaps I should say fastest, highest, strongest), and it doesn't matter who or where the person is.

Presumably, psychology's unique domain is the individual; understanding who the person is is the essence of psychology's contribution, but we do little to individualize our work. We could start with the perspective of the performer and determine the meaning of enhanced performance or excellence for that individual before we try to figure out how to enhance performance or achieve excellence.

Some of the sport and exercise psychology research that we do have, as Dan discussed, points out the importance of individualized interventions. For example, the most recent research and theory on anxiety and sport performance (see Gould & Krane, in press, for a current review of that work) emphasizes individual measures, anxiety patterns, and interventions. That is, what works for one person does not necessarily work for another, or even for that same person in a different situation or at a different time. Most applied sport psychologists who work with athletes now attempt to individualize performance enhancement techniques and programs.

We could take individualization much further. Rather than assume the same performance standards for all, we could individualize performance standards. We typically assume that everyone on a track team focuses on running faster or placing higher, but that may not be the case. Moreover, within sport and exercise psychology, we now recognize that an emphasis on *performance* rather than on outcomes is a better approach.

But, even with a performance focus (versus a win or outcome focus) we seldom consider the individual. For example, my biomechanics colleague (Hudson, in press) argues that we could assess excellence in the 100-m dash by calculating relative velocities as the distance in height divided by the elapsed time, rather than simply as time over the 100 m. Hudson's calculation would individualize performance relative to one relevant individual characteristic: height.

From that perspective, Carl Lewis, who stands 6′2″ tall and set the men's world record of 9.92 seconds at the Seoul Olympics in 1988, has a relative velocity of 5.36 heights per second. Florence Griffith-Joyner, the women's winner at Seoul, is 5′6-1/2″ tall, ran the 100 m in 10.49 seconds, and has a relative velocity of 5.64 heights per second. Who is the fastest human? We could use many different characteristics, and this is just one example. The point is that, by taking different individual standards, we arrive at different standards of excellence, different performance enhancement goals, and different strategies for reaching those goals.

From a sport psychology perspective, we could go further and consider the individual in more than biomechanical and physiological terms. We could also individualize standards of excellence and approaches in terms of a wider range of individual capabilities, interests, goals, and especially in relation to their sociocultural context (as Sage and Harris discuss in their papers in this volume).

This type of individualization gets into another limitation for sport psychology's performance enhancement work. My emphasis and perspective within sport and exercise psychology differs from Dan's in that I place more emphasis on social context. Generally, I see psychology as a behavioral science that focuses on the individual and fits between biological and social sciences. Within sport and exercise science, sport and exercise psychology makes its strongest contribution when it is informed by both biological and social science perspectives. So we need more than a psychobiological perspective; we need a biopsychosocial perspective, with sport and exercise psychology in the middle focusing on the whole individual.

Many sociocultural scholars, especially those not trained in physical education, dismiss biological factors and processes. Certainly this is a limitation; if we want to understand human behavior in physical activity contexts, we cannot dismiss the physical. But I also believe that if we ignore the wide range of individual differences and isolate movement or activity from its sociocultural context, we no longer have human behavior. In the recent past, sport psychology has moved too far away from sociocultural areas and lost much of its real value.

Sport and exercise psychology is a behavioral science (or perhaps an art), and our proper focus is on behavior. We might incorporate specific biological or sociocultural factors, but to understand behavior we should focus on behavior in a holistic sense and not on component parts or isolated determinants. When we break behavior down into component parts and strip away the sociocultural context, we no longer have behavior—and all the sophisticated MANOVA and LISREL programs won't put Humpty Dumpty back together.

Some have suggested that we should abandon quantitative analyses and the scientific approach to get back to sport behavior. I do not think that is necessarily the way to go, although sport psychology could benefit by incorporating more interpretive analyses and qualitative information. I believe the main issue is the focus of study and not how we measure. That is, the focus should be on behavior, and we might work on developing appropriate behavioral measures and analyses, whether they are quantitative or qualitative.

One approach I find intriguing at the moment is the dynamical systems or chaos theory approach that is being incorporated in some of our motor behavior work (e.g., Clark & Whitall, 1989; Kelso & Tuller, 1984) as well as in varied other fields from physics to economics. For example, a recent compilation by the American Association for the Advancement of Science (Krasner, 1990) documented the application of chaos to biological processes including brain electrical activity and heart rhythms, business and economics, and epidemiology, as well as to physical systems.

Social science, and specifically social psychology, has been slower to incorporate dynamical systems, but Richter (1986) specifically suggests treating social behavior as nonlinear behavior with chaos theory models. Given my limited understanding based on cursory readings of chaos theory (Gleick, 1987) and discussions with motor behavior colleagues, I have only a general impression of dynamical systems and a vague idea of how we might apply it to sport psychology. The main aspect of chaos that appeals to me, at least with my understanding, is the recognition that precise, linear predictions are not possible—even if we continue to refine our measures and multivariate designs.

If chaos theorists suggest that it is impossible to predict the weather, certainly it seems unlikely that we will predict sport performance. If butterfly wings can alter weather patterns, certainly many "little" things—the comment from the elementary physical education teacher, the parents' reaction to backyard baseball, the placement of mirrors in the exercise room, or the attitude of your supervisor at work—can affect sport and exercise performance somehow at some time. We might better look at behavior in a more holistic sense, over time and conditions, and try to find patterns rather than search for minor fluctuations in behavior or performance.

Sport psychology might contribute more to performance enhancement if we abandoned the search for more complete linear, predictive models and attempted to describe behavior *patterns*. We might look at variations in patterns across individuals—the Olympic athlete, the 10-year-old, or the adult jogger—or how patterns vary over time and conditions within an individual. Although descriptive work seems to be second class in our research hierarchy, we might help more individuals find their own standard of excellence as well as find more ways to enhance performance with this approach.

References

Clark, J.E., & Whitall, J. (1989). What is motor development? The lessons of history. *Quest*, **41**, 183-202.

Feltz, D.L., & Landers, D.M. (1983). The effects of mental practice on motor skill learning and performance: A meta-analysis. *Journal of Sport Psychology*, **5**, 25-57.

Gleick, J. (1987). *Chaos: The making of a new science*. New York: Viking.

Gould, D., & Krane, V. (in press). The anxiety-athletic performance relationship: Current status and future directions. In T. Horn (Ed.), *Advances in sport psychology*. Champaign, IL: Human Kinetics.

Hudson, J.L. (in press). It's mostly a matter of metric. In D.M. Costa & S.R. Guthrie (Eds.), *Women and sport*. Champaign, IL: Human Kinetics.

Kelso, J.A.S., & Tuller, B. (1984). A dynamical basis for action systems. In M. Gazzaniga (Ed.), *Handbook of cognitive neuroscience* (pp. 321-356). New York: Plenum.

Krasner, S. (Ed.) (1990). *The ubiquity of chaos*. Washington, DC: American Association for the Advancement of Science.

Landers, D.M. (in press). Sport psychology techniques to optimize the preparation to perform under pressure. In R. Bjork & D. Druckman (Eds.), *In the mind's eye: Understanding human performance*. Washington, DC: National Academy Press.

Richter, F.M. (1986). Non-linear behavior. In D.W. Fiske & R.A. Shewder (Eds.), *Metatheory in social science* (pp. 284-292). Chicago: University of Chicago Press.

Application of Exercise Physiology to the Enhancement of Human Performance

James S. Skinner
Arizona State University

Before beginning this paper, it is important to point out that few innovative studies or major new ideas have emerged in the recent past relative to applying knowledge about exercise physiology to enhance performance. More often it has been a matter of refining what is already known and applying this knowledge to other situations. A good example of this is the knowledge about carbohydrate (CHO) loading. Christensen and Hansen first suggested in 1939 that a high CHO diet enhances endurance exercise performance.

After this basic research was redone in a more sophisticated manner two decades later by Bergstrom, Hermansen, Hultman, and Saltin (1967), and publicized, CHO loading became the thing to do among marathon runners. There were many problems associated with depletion of muscle glycogen stores, however, and more recent studies have demonstrated that it is not necessary to exhaust muscle glycogen if one trains regularly, consumes a high CHO diet, and rests a few days before competition (Costill, 1986).

Scientists and practitioners (e.g., physical educators, fitness professionals, and coaches) also may not be aware of what was done before they became interested in a problem or a field of study. As an example, today's "new" programs of low-impact aerobics are not much different from the rhythmical, continuous calisthenics done by knowledgeable physical educators 40–50 years ago (Skinner, 1987).

Scientists and practitioners rarely communicate. When they do, they use different jargon and may neither trust nor understand one another. As a result, some practitioners use hit-or-miss approaches that ignore the findings of research. On the other hand, some exercise scientists attempt to explain why the empirical findings of particular practitioners are successful (i.e., why their methods work), but they do not always do a good job of relaying the information back to those practitioners in a way that is understandable and useful.

While it is highly unlikely that this paper will have a significant effect on this gap, it will attempt to summarize some findings in several areas of exercise physiology and discuss briefly whether and how these findings might enhance exercise performance.

Basic Principles

There are two main principles related to training and enhancement of exercise performance. The *overload* principle states that a system must be overloaded or stimulated adequately for structural or functional adaptations to occur. More important for enhancing performance is the principle of *specificity*, which states that adaptations are specific to the various systems and their structural and functional elements that are overloaded (i.e., adaptations occur only in those systems adequately stimulated). As an example, weightlifting is a brief, high-intensity, anaerobic (AN) exercise stimulating the skeletal and neuromuscular systems whereas marathon running is a prolonged, low-intensity, aerobic (AER) activity that stimulates those systems involved in the transport and utilization of oxygen.

Specific training effects can be seen even in athletes who appear to stimulate the same systems. For example, swimmers, runners, and cyclists all have good endurance and a high maximal AER power ($\dot{V}O_2$max). However, each will perform best in his or her particular activity. On the other hand, triathletes train with all three modes of exercise and tend to have $\dot{V}O_2$max values in each activity that are halfway between those typically seen in untrained people and those from athletes who train specifically in only one of the three activities (Kohrt, O'Connor, & Skinner, 1987). It is this factor of specificity that makes studying the physiology of exercise and training so complex, challenging, and interesting.

It is a basic principle of exercise physiology that a given power output requires a given amount of energy, regardless of the mechanism by which that energy is produced. Some energy is immediately available in the muscle in a form (ATP and PC) that can be used anaerobically, especially when energy is needed rapidly such as at the onset of more intense exercise.

High-intensity, short-duration, and static exercise tends to be primarily AN. Only CHO is used for fuel, and lactate (LA) is produced when this fast, less efficient "backup system" is used. Low-intensity, prolonged, and dynamic exercise, on the other hand, tends to be primarily AER; this is a slower, more efficient system which uses "unlimited" supplies of stored CHO and fats.

From the description of the three broad classifications of exercise given above, it can be seen that the relative contribution of AER and AN energy production depends on the type, intensity, and duration of exercise and that intensity and duration of exercise are inversely related. *Aerobic* activities requiring less than 50% $\dot{V}O_2$max can generally be done for ≥ 8 hours, whereas those AER activities requiring <90% but >65% $\dot{V}O_2$max can be done from 10 minutes to 2 hours, respectively. When activities require <200% but >90–95% $\dot{V}O_2$max, they are a mixture of AN and AER exercise, can be sustained from 1 to 8 min, respectively, and are associated with the highest levels of blood LA. *Anaerobic* activities are those whose energy requirement is <450%, but >200% $\dot{V}O_2$max, and which can be done from 1 to 45 sec, respectively. For more detailed information on these classifications, the reader is referred to reviews by Skinner and Morgan (1985) and Skinner, Noeldner, and O'Connor (1989).

Specificity of Different Types of Training Programs

Wilmore and Costill (1988) reported on the specific effects of AER (30-min bouts) and AN (6-sec and 30-sec bouts) training on the enzymes associated with the various energy systems in muscle. They found that 30-sec AN training signifi-cantly increased the enzymes associated with ATP resynthesis but not the 6-sec bouts (probably because the stimulus was too brief to be effective). Only the 30-sec bouts significantly increased the activity of the glycolytic enzymes. As expected, the largest increases in oxidative enzyme activity occurred with 30-min AER training, although there was a smaller but significant rise with 30-sec training bouts. These findings suggest that 30-sec interval AN training programs can improve all three energy-producing systems.

Skinner and O'Connor (1987) did a cross-sectional study on five groups of athletes who train differently. There were two AN groups (powerlifters and gymnasts), one AER–AN group (wrestlers), and two AER groups (10-km runners and ultramarathoners). Using the Wingate Test to measure AN ability, it was found that powerlifters had a significantly higher 5-sec peak power output (PO) compared to ultramarathoners. The other athletes were distributed in a logical order, based on their type of training.

Interestingly, there was no difference among the athletes in the mean 30-sec PO. This was explained by the fact that AN athletes started with higher values but had a faster rate of fatigue, while AER athletes had lower initial values and less of a decrement over the 30-sec test. This is probably associated with the different muscle fiber compositions and different training programs of these athletes.

As a continuation of this study, Skinner and O'Connor (1987) also performed a training study using five different programs. Subjects trained

1. 10 sec at a PO requiring about 240% $\dot{V}O_2$max alternating with 30 sec rest for 40 min (AN);
2. 30 sec at a PO requiring about 180% $\dot{V}O_2$max alternating with 90 sec rest for 40 min (AN);
3. 2 min at 120% $\dot{V}O_2$max alternating with 6 min rest for 40 min (AER–AN);
4. 30 min at 80% $\dot{V}O_2$max (AER); or
5. 60 min at 60% $\dot{V}O_2$max (AER).

Results from the Wingate Test showed that the 10-sec AN program produced a significant rise in peak 5-sec PO, the 30-sec AN program caused a significant increase in 30-sec mean PO, and the 2-min AER–AN program improved both peak 5-sec and mean 30-sec values. The AER programs had little effect on AN measures, reaffirming the specificty principle. Interestingly, all five programs produced a signficant rise in $\dot{V}O_2$max. The unexpected rise in maximal aerobic power from the AN programs is probably due to the fact that the rest intervals were too short to allow the aerobic system to return to baseline before the next exercise interval began. These suggestive findings agree with those by Wilmore and Costill (1988) mentioned above, that high-intensity interval training programs can improve all three energy systems.

Other Factors Associated With Exercise Performance

Brief, High-Intensity Exercise

High levels of blood LA are found with AN activities lasting 1–8 min (Skinner & Morgan, 1985). Using athletes whose sporting event lasted from 1 to 8 min,

Mader, Heck, and Hollman (1978) had them run or swim the same distance as for their competitive events but at several submaximal speeds. These speeds were designed to produce blood LA levels above 4 mM but below those seen in competition. Because of a linear relationship between LA and speed at these intensities, they could extrapolate LA values to the maximal levels obtained after competition and estimate the maximal speed at which the athlete should be able to perform.

These results were then used to control training intensity and to estimate the effects of training without having the athlete perform maximally. Thus, if an athlete improved, LA at a given speed dropped and the parallel line would shift to the right, suggesting that the athlete could run or swim faster at the same maximal LA. Conversely, if the athlete was overtrained, LA at a given speed would increase, the line would shift to the left, and training could be adjusted. This method has been used successfully to train many athletes.

Because high-intensity exercise lasting 1–8 min increases the concentrations of LA and hydrogen ions (H^+) in blood and muscle, and because these high levels of acidity adversely affect energy production, there have been numerous attempts to reduce acidity with buffers, especially sodium bicarbonate. This compound is used because it is thought to delay fatigue by increasing the gradient and diffusion rate of LA and H^+ from muscle to blood (Mainwood & Cechetto, 1980).

While there have been conflicting results, a recent study by Horswill et al. (1988) found that the total work output in 2 min did not differ when subjects were given 0, 10, 15, and 20 gm $NaHCO_3$ per kg body weight, even though plasma HCO_3^- levels were higher and related to the dosage given. Reviewing other studies, Horswill et al. (1988) concluded that bicarbonate loading might be effective if higher dosages (e.g., >30 gm/kg) and/or repeated bouts of near-maximal exercise were studied. Nevertheless, many subjects have gastrointestinal distress and diarrhea within 1 hour of ingestion, which suggests that taking bicarbonate is not a practical way to improve performance of this type of exercise.

Prolonged, Moderate-Intensity Exercise

Much more is known about prolonged, moderate-intensity AER exercise than brief, high-intensity AN exercise. First, it is easier to study AER exercise because the subject reaches a steady state at which there is little change in physiological parameters of interest. This is not the case with brief AN exercise, in which technique and motivation are often more important. Prolonged exercise also offers a good model for studying the responses and adaptations of the cardiovascular, respiratory, nervous, muscular, endocrine, and thermoregulatory systems, as well as the effect of nutrition. High-intensity AN exercise, on the other hand, involves primarily the nervous and muscular systems.

There is a controversy about which variables should be used to predict performance of this type of exercise. Although a high $\dot{V}O_2max$ is an important and necessary factor in one's ability to compete successfully in endurance events, it is not the main determinant of success once high values are reached. For example, Costill (1986) reported that $\dot{V}O_2max$ is not predictive of success when a homogeneous group of endurance athletes compete with one another, as is generally the case.

While $\dot{V}O_2max$ is associated with endurance capacity, defined as the ability to sustain a high percentage of $\dot{V}O_2max$ for a prolonged period, the two are not closely related (Bouchard & Lortie, 1984; Péronnet, Thibault, Rhodes, & McKenzie, 1987). Thus, a high $\dot{V}O_2$max is needed to perform well, but good endurance performance is also associated with

- A high percentage of Type I (slow-twitch) muscle fibers;
- Ability to store muscle and liver glycogen;
- Ability to use free fatty acids, thus sparing limited glycogen stores;
- Ability to sustain a high percentage of one's $\dot{V}O_2$max;
- Economy of movement; and
- Ability to dissipate body heat.

Percentage of Type I Muscle Fibers. With a richer supply of capillaries to bring oxygen and substrates and a higher density of mitochondria to provide energy aerobically, Type I fibers are more fatigue resistant than Type II (fast-twitch) fibers. Although it has been shown that a higher precentage of Type I fibers is associated with a greater endurance ability, fiber composition alone is not a reliable predictor of endurance performance (Wilmore & Costill, 1988). The fatigue-resistant characteristics of the Type I fibers can be enhanced by endurance training, but the percentage of the various fiber types is not altered (Wilmore & Costill, 1988).

Ability to Store Muscle and Liver Glycogen. Given that the body always uses CHO and that it has limited glycogen stores, it is logical that good endurance is associated with the ability to store high levels of glycogen in the main reservoirs, muscle and liver. As mentioned earlier, the classic manner for increasing the amount of glycogen stored in the body is CHO loading or supercompensation of muscle glycogen (Bergstrom et al., 1967).

However, given that (a) high glycogen stores are not critical except in endurance events lasting more than 60–90 min (Saltin, 1975); (b) training is perceived to be more difficult and there is a greater risk of injury when glycogen stores are depleted (Wilmore & Costill, 1988); and (c) regular endurance training and a high CHO diet can maintain higher than normal muscle glycogen levels (Wilmore & Costill, 1988), CHO loading may not be needed. Reducing the intensity and duration of training in the week before competition and eating a high CHO diet appears to be as effective, without the psychological problems.

Ability to Use Free Fatty Acids (FFA). In addition to increasing glycogen stores in the body, reducing the use of CHO is also associated with good endurance. One approach has been to take caffeine 1 hour before competition (Costill, Dalsky, & Fink, 1978) to stimulate the release of FFA and increase the utilization of fat for energy. The effects of caffeine ingestion are not always successful, however, and some people have such negative side effects as diuresis and cardiac arrhythmias. Of greater importance for conserving limited glycogen stores is the improved ability of muscle to use fat as a result of endurance training. Well-trained endurance athletes have a higher density of capillaries and mitochondria and an increased activity of those enzymes involved in fat oxidation (Holloszy & Booth, 1976).

Ability to Sustain a High Pecentage of One's $\dot{V}O_2$max. Péronnet et al. (1987) define endurance capability as the ability to sustain a high fraction of $\dot{V}O_2$max for a prolonged time and found that it was closely related to the %$\dot{V}O_2$max at the ventilatory threshold. This agrees with the findings of McLellan and Skinner (1985) that time to fatigue was significantly longer in persons of high and medium fitness than in those with low levels of fitness (mean $\dot{V}O_2$max values were 58.3, 50.5, and 41.8 ml•kg^{-1}•min^{-1}, respectively). They also found that expressing the intensity of exercise relative to ventilatory thresholds reduced the standard error of estimate for predicting endurance times by 30% compared with using %$\dot{V}O_2$max, the usual method for expressing exercise intensity.

Although there is a controversy about how to measure the various thresholds, their possible physiological significance, and what mechanisms are responsible for them, it is generally accepted that endurance athletes tend to have higher thresholds (Svedenhag & Sjödin, 1984), that these thresholds can be elevated by endurance training (Wilmore & Costill, 1988), and that running speed or absolute power output at the threshold is a good predictor of endurance performance (Péronnet et al., 1987).

Economy of Movement. The ability to use less energy while moving at the same speed is an obvious advantage in many sports. Among runners with similar $\dot{V}O_2$max values, much of the variation in distance running performance can be explained by differences in running economy (Daniels, 1985). A number of studies have shown that marathoners run more economically (i.e., they use 5–10% less energy) than runners trained for shorter distances (Costill, 1986).

Whether the different economy of movement is related to body structure and its associated mechanical constraints or to the type and amount of training is not known. Indeed, it is not clear whether training can modify economy in those who have competed for a number of years. The substantial variation in economy among endurance athletes suggests that nontraining factors are important (Morgan, Martin, Krahenbuhl, & Baldini, 1991).

Ability to Dissipate Body Heat. Regular endurance training produces a partial acclimatization to heat because of the higher body temperature during long training sessions (Gisolfi & Robinson, 1969). Endurance athletes sweat more and sooner than untrained persons, effectively keeping their temperature lower during prolonged exercise (Nadel, 1988). This lower temperature is associated with a reduced blood flow to the skin, resulting in a greater flow to transport oxygen and nutrients to working muscles. Endurance athletes also have a greater blood volume, which gives them a greater resistance to heat syncope than untrained, unacclimatized persons (Nadel, 1988).

Genetics and Trainability

Studies by Bouchard and his colleagues indicate that genetics play an important role in the response to training. There are large individual differences in the ability to train one's AER and AN abilities. For example, while mean training gains in AER ability ($\dot{V}O_2$max and maximal work output in 90 min) were 33 and 51%, respectively, the variation in gains ranged from 10 to 90%. Anaerobic ability (maximal work outputs in 10 sec and 90 sec) improved an average of 22 and 35%, respectively, ranging from 5 to 70% (Bouchard, Boulay, Simoneau, Lortie, & Pérusse, 1988). These values are typical of what has been found in other studies (Dionne et al., 1991). Data from many studies also suggest that there are low responders and high responders, as well as those who respond early and those who respond late to training.

The size of the genetic effect is about 40% for $\dot{V}O_2$max (ml•kg^{-1}•min^{-1}) and 60–70% for the 90-min total work output, that is, the effect is greater for endurance performance than for maximal aerobic power (Bouchard et al., 1988).

The difference in response to endurance training is 65–80% genotype dependent, especially in the latter stages of long-term training when subjects approach their genetic limits of adaptation (Hamel, Simoneau, Lortie, Boulay, & Bouchard, 1986). Simoneau et al. (1986) looked at the genetic effect on training responses to brief AN exercise (10-sec work output) and to longer AN exercise (90-sec work output). The genetic effect was low (30%) for the 10-sec exercise but significant (70%) for the 90-sec bout.

Summary

Many factors mentioned in this paper may be influenced by genetics and training and are often interrelated. For example, a high $\dot{V}O_2$max and the ability to perform at a high percentage of one's $\dot{V}O_2$max can be influenced by training and heredity. It is not known whether economy of movement is similarly affected. Training and diet both affect the ability to store more CHO and to use more fat; this is also influenced by muscle fiber composition, which has a strong genetic influence. Muscle fiber composition is also an important factor in the performance of brief, high-intensity AN exercise.

As a result of endurance training, body weight and body fat are reduced. This lowers heat production, decreases the insulating effect of subcutaneous fat, and improves the ability to dissipate body heat. The expanded blood volume associated with a greater resistance to heat syncope is also associated with a higher $\dot{V}O_2$max. Because of all these possible interrelationships, therefore, it is not possible to select any one factor as the most important for the ability to perform any type of exercise on the continuum from low-intensity, prolonged AER exercise to high-intensity, brief AN exercise.

Given the present state of knowledge, it is not possible to accurately predict the response of any individual to a given training stimulus. It appears that very high levels of AN and/or AER performance are the result of having (a) the right ancestors, (b) an adequate program of training, rest, and nutrition, and (c) genetic characteristics associated with high-responder status.

References

Bergstrom, J., Hermansen, L., Hultman, E., & Saltin, B. (1967). Diet, muscle glycogen, and physical performance. *Acta Physiologica Scandinavica*, **71**, 140-150.

Bouchard, C., Boulay, M.R., Simoneau, J.-A., Lortie, G., & Pérusse, L. (1988). Heredity and trainability of aerobic and anaerobic performances. An update. *Sports Medicine*, **5**, 69-73.

Bouchard, C., & Lortie, G. (1984). Heredity and endurance performance. *Sports Medicine*, **1**, 38-64.

Christensen, E.H., & Hansen, O. (1939). Zur Methodik der respiratorischen Quotient-Bestimmung in Ruhe und bei Arbeit [On the method of respiratory quotient determination at rest and during work]. *Skandinavische Archiv für Physiologie*, **81**, 137-143.

Costill, D.L. (1986). *Inside running: Basics of sports physiology*. Indianapolis: Benchmark Press.

Costill, D.L., Dalsky, G.P., & Fink, W.J. (1978). Effects of caffeine ingestion on metabolism and exercise performance. *Medicine and Science in Sports and Exercise*, **10**, 155-158.

Daniels, J. (1985). A physiologist's view of running economy. *Medicine and Science in Sports and Exercise*, **17**, 332-338.

Dionne, F.T., Turcotte, L., Thibault, M.C., Boulay, M.R., Skinner, J.S., & Bouchard, C. (1991). Mitochondrial DNA sequence polymorphism, $\dot{V}O_2$max, and response to endurance training. *Medicine and Science in Sports and Exercise*, **23**, 177-185.

Gisolfi, C., & Robinson, S. (1969). Relations between physical training, acclimatization and heat tolerance. *Journal of Applied Physiology*, **26**, 530-534.

Hamel, P., Simoneau, J.A., Lortie, G., Boulay, M.R., & Bouchard, C. (1986). Heredity and muscle adaptation to endurance training. *Medicine and Science in Sports and Exercise*, **18**, 690-696.

Holloszy, J.O., & Booth, F.W. (1976). Biochemical adaptations to endurance exercise in muscle. *Annual Reveiw of Physiology*, **18**, 273-291.

Horswill, C.A., Costill, D.L., Fink, W.J., Flynn, M.G., Kirwan, J.P., Mitchell, J.B., & Houmard, J.A. (1988). Influence of sodium bicarbonate on sprint performance: Relationship to dosage. *Medicine and Science in Sports and Exercise*, **20**, 566-569.

Kohrt, W.M., O'Connor, J.S., & Skinner, J.S. (1987). Physiological responses of triathletes to maximal swimming, cycling and running. *Medicine and Science in Sports and Exercise*, **19**, 51-55.

Mader, A., Heck, H., & Hollmann, W. (1978). Evaluation of lactic acid anaerobic energy contribution by determination of postexercise lactic acid concentration of ear capillary blood in middle-distance runners and swimmers. In F. Landry & W. Orban (Eds.), *The International Congress of Physical Activity Sciences* (Vol. 4). Exercise Physiology. Miami: Symposium Specialists.

Mainwood, G.W., & Cechetto, D. (1980). The effect of bicarbonate concentration on fatigue and recovery in isolated rat diaphragm. *Canadian Journal of Physiology and Pharmacology*, **58**, 624-632.

McLellan, T.M., & Skinner, J.S. (1985). Submaximal endurance performance related to the ventilzation thresholds. *Canadian Journal of Applied Sports Sciences*, **10**, 81-87.

Morgan, D.W., Martin, P.E., Krahenbuhl, G.S., & Baldini, F.D. (1991). Variability in running economy and mechanics among trained male runners. *Medicine and Science in Sports and Exercise*, **23**, 378-383.

Nadel, E.R. (1988). Temperature regulation and prolonged exercise. In D.R. Lamb & R. Murray (Eds.), *Perspectives in exercise science and sports medicine. Volume I: Prolonged exercise* (pp. 125-152). Indianapolis: Benchmark Press.

Péronnet, F., Thibault, G., Rhodes, E.C., & McKenzie, D.C. (1987). Correlation between ventilatory threshold and endurance capability in marathon runners. *Medicine and Science in Sports and Exercise*, **19**, 610-615.

Saltin, B. (1975). Adaptive changes in carbohydrate metabolism with exercise. In H. Howald & J. Poortmans (Eds.), *Metabolic adaptation to prolonged physical exercise* (pp. 94-100). Basel: Birkhäuser Verlag.

Simoneau, J.A., Lortie, G., Boulay, M.R., Marcotte, M., Thibault, M.C., & Bouchard, C. (1986). Inheritance of human skeletal muscle and anaerobic capacity adaptation to high-intensity intermittent training. *International Journal of Sports Medicine*, **7**, 167-171.

Skinner, J.S. (1987). The fitness industry. In R.M. Malina & H.M. Eckert (Eds.), The Academy Papers (No. 21) *Physical activity in early and modern populations* (pp. 67-72). Champaign, IL: Human Kinetics.

Skinner, J.S., & Morgan, D.W. (1985). Aspects of anaerobic performance. In D.H. Clarke & H.M. Eckert (Eds.), The Academy Papers (No. 18) Limits of human performance (pp. 31-44). Champaign, IL: Human Kinetics.

Skinner, J.S., Noeldner, S.P., & O'Connor, J.S. (1989). The development and maintenance of physical fitness. In A.J. Ryan & F.L. Allman (Eds.), *Sports medicine* (2nd ed., pp. 515-528). New York: Academic Press.

Skinner, J.S., & O'Connor, J.S. (1987). Wingate test — Cross-sectional and longitudinal analysis. *Medicine and Science in Sports and Exercise*, **19**, S73.

Svedenhag, J., & Sjödin, B. (1984). Maximal and submaximal oxygen uptakes and blood lactate levels in elite male middle- and long-distance runners. *International Journal of Sports Medicine*, **5**, 255-261.

Wilmore, J.H., & Costill, D.L. (1988). *Training for sport and activity* (3rd ed.). Dubuque, IA: Wm. C. Brown.

Application of Exercise Physiology to the Enhancement of Human Performance —Reaction

Emily M. Haymes
Florida State University

There are many applications of exercise physiology that have been used to enhance performance in sports. The preceding paper by Skinner has outlined some of the most important applications of training for improving performance. One concept that has attracted considerable research interest is that nutrition can enhance performance. Much of this interest has focused on carbohydrate ingestion prior to and during exercise as well as the need to replenish carbohydrates following exercise.

Carbohydrate Ingestion and Performance

The concept of carbohydrate loading for several days prior to endurance events has been well accepted both by the scientific community and by coaches and athletes for many years. Meals that are high in carbohydrate (70% or more of the total calories) are consumed for 2 to 3 days while the athlete tapers training immediately prior to competition (Sherman, Costill, Fink, & Miller, 1981). Muscle glycogen concentration increases to levels well above normal after 48 hours of carbohydrate loading. This dietary manipulation is most effective in events that last 2 hours or more (Karlsson & Saltin, 1971).

Whether the meal immediately prior to competition should be high in carbohydrates has been the subject of several recent investigations. Subjects who consumed 75 grams of glucose 45 minutes prior to exercise experienced low blood glucose concentrations after 20 minutes of exercise (Costill et al., 1977). Glucose ingestion and subsequent absorption into the blood stimulates an insulin response prior to exercise. When exercise begins, insulin accelerates the uptake of glucose by the tissues.

In a subsequent study, Foster, Costill, and Fink (1979) found that glucose feeding 30 minutes prior to exercise reduced endurance at 80% $\dot{V}O_2$max even though blood glucose was not significantly lower than the control treatment at exhaustion. In order to avoid an insulin response, it has been suggested that carbohydrate meals should be ingested 3-4 hours before exercise. Ingestion of a high carbohydrate meal 4 hours before exercise resulted in lower blood glucose concentrations during the first hour of exercise, but also increased muscle glycogen stores prior to exercise (Coyle, Coggan, Hemmert, Lowe, & Walters, 1985).

The combination of a light carbohydrate meal (200 g CHO) 4 hours before exercise plus a confectionery bar (45 g CHO) 5 minutes before exercise significantly increased the total amount of work done on a cycle ergometer (Neufer et al., 1987). Eating the confectionery bar or consuming a carbohydrate drink 5 minutes before exercise produced more work than the fasting state, but neither was as effective as the light carbohydrate meal/confectionery bar combination.

Carbohydrate feeding during exercise may be beneficial in improving performance in prolonged exercise events. Dilute carbohydrate solutions (<10% CHO) are used during exercise because more concentrated solutions delay gastric emptying. Trained cyclists were better able to maintain blood glucose for 180 minutes of exercise if they consumed a glucose polymer solution periodically during exercise at 75% $\dot{V}O_2$max rather than a placebo (Coyle et al., 1983). Fatigue occurred earlier in the placebo trial.

Wilber (1990) found that distance runners could run longer at 80% $\dot{V}O_2$max if they drank a glucose polymer solution at 15-min intervals instead of an artificially sweetened drink. The beneficial effect of carbohydrate replacement during exercise may be intensity specific. There was no significant difference in time to exhaustion during cycling at 85% $\dot{V}O_2$max between glucose polymer, placebo, and electrolyte drinks (Powers et al., 1990). The length of the cycling bout (40 minutes) would not be sufficient to deplete muscle glycogen stores. Carbohydrate replacement during exercise is most likely to be beneficial in events lasting 90 minutes or more.

Muscle glycogen is gradually depleted when athletes train over consecutive days unless adequate carbohydrate is included in the diet (Costill, Bowers, Branam, & Sparks, 1971). Diets that contain 70% of the total calories as carbohydrate result in more glycogen being stored in the muscles than diets that are 50% carbohydrate, the typical American diet (Costill et al., 1981). Muscle glycogen synthesis is greater if carbohydrates are eaten immediately following exercise rather than 2 hours later (Ivy, Katz, Cutler, Sherman, & Coyle, 1988). "Therefore, to maximize muscle glycogen synthesis following exercise, athletes should ingest high carbohydrate beverages and snacks as soon as possible following a strenuous workout or competition," say Sherman and Wimer (1991, p. 32).

Blood Volume Changes and Performance

Another concept that has intrigued exercise physiologists, coaches, and athletes is that changes in blood volume can alter performance. Blood volume is subdivided into two fractions: cellular volume (mostly red blood cells or erythrocytes) and plasma volume. Red blood cells are the primary carrier of oxygen to the tissues. Expansion of the red cell volume should increase performance in aerobic endurance sports because more oxygen will be delivered to the muscles. There are several ways that red blood cell volume can be expanded: living at high altitudes, red cell infusion (blood doping), and use of erythropoietin.

Expansion of red cell volume begins almost immediately when a person goes to high altitude, but it is accompanied initially by a reduction in plasma volume so that total blood volume remains relatively constant. After 2 months at altitude, red cell volume expansion increases total blood volume (Reynafarje, Lozano, & Valdivieso, 1959). Expansion of red cell volume is accompanied by increases in $\dot{V}O_2$max and endurance at altitude (Horstman, Weiskopf, & Jackson, 1980).

Some world class runners and cyclists choose to live and train at altitude in the hope of gaining a competitive advantage from the expanded red cell volume.

Reinfusion of a person's own red blood cells will expand the red cell volume and increase $\dot{V}O_2$max and endurance (Buick, Gledhill, Froese, & Spriet, 1982). Usually two pints of blood are removed from the subject and stored in a blood bank for 6 weeks or longer, then the red blood cells are reinfused. Highly trained distance runners ran 5 miles significantly faster following red blood cell infusion than when saline was infused (Williams, Wesseldine, Somma, & Schuster, 1981).

At the 1984 Olympics, eight members of the U.S. Cycling Team were involved in a scheme to improve performance by infusing red blood cells. In some cases athletes were infusing other people's blood, which can be dangerous because of the risk of infection. Both the International Olympic Committee and the U.S. Olympic Committee in 1985 banned infusion of blood by athletes as unethical (Caldwell & Jopke, 1985). At the present time, however, it is not possible to detect whether a person has reinfused his or her own red blood cells.

The newest technique for expanding red cell volume is the use of erythropoietin, a hormone produced by the kidneys that stimulates the red bone marrow to form red blood cells. In 1989 the Food and Drug Administration approved the use of erythropoietin, which was intended for use in kidney patients who do not form the natural hormone. Erythropoietin will increase red cell volume in 5–10 days.

It appears that some athletes may be using erythropoietin to expand their red cell volume. This could be dangerous if erythropoietin is used too often: Expansion of red cell volume to abnormally high levels (polycythemia) increases resistance to blood flow and leads to blood clotting. The risk of heart attack and stroke is greater in persons with polycythemia.

Expansion of plasma volume may also improve performance. Plasma volume can be increased by using plasma volume expanders (e.g., 5% serum albumin, isotonic saline) or by training. When athletes begin training, there is approximately a 15% increase in plasma volume over the first few weeks of training. Detraining produces a gradual loss of plasma volume. The primary advantage of an expanded plasma volume appears to be better maintenance of blood flow to the skin and central blood volume during exercise in warm environments (Nose, Mack, Shi, Morimoto, & Nadel, 1990).

Although expanding the red cell volume improves oxygen transport to the tissues, reducing red cell volume, as occurs in anemia, limits oxygen transport to the tissues. If the anemia is due to iron deficiency, tissue iron depletion may also be present. Anemia significantly lowers $\dot{V}O_2$max and endurance (Celsing, Blomstrand, Werner, Pihlstedt, & Ekblom, 1986). Tissue iron depletion can also impair aerobic performance because many mitochondrial enzymes have iron as part of their structure (Davies, Maguire, Brooks, Dallman, & Packer, 1982). Use of iron supplements by women athletes who are iron deficient but not anemic will improve iron status and may improve endurance (Rowland, Deisroth, Green, & Kelleher, 1988).

Conclusion

The concept that carbohydrate ingestion can enhance performance is applicable to many sports and all levels of training and competition. The concept that blood volume increases can enhance performance has been most widely used and abused by elite endurance athletes. The concept that decreases in red cell volume and tissue iron depletion can impair performance has broad application to women athletes competing in many sports.

References

Buick, F.J., Gledhill, N., Froese, A., & Spriet, L.L. (1982). Red cell mass and aerobic performance at sea level. In J.R. Sutton, N.L. Jones, & C.S. Houston (Eds.), *Hypoxia: Man at altitude* (pp. 43-50). New York: Thieme-Stratton.

Caldwell, F., & Jopke, T. (1985). Questions and answers: ACSM 1985. *The Physician and Sportsmedicine*, **13**(8), 145-151.

Celsing, F., Blomstrand, E., Werner, B., Pihlstedt, P., & Ekblom, B. (1986). Effects of iron deficiency on endurance and muscle enzyme activity in man. *Medicine and Science in Sports and Exercise*, **18**, 156-161.

Costill, D.L., Bowers, R., Branam, G., & Sparks, K. (1971). Muscle glycogen utilization during prolonged exercise on successive days. *Journal of Applied Physiology*, **31**, 834-838.

Costill, D.L., Coyle, E., Dalsky, G., Evans, W., Fink, W., & Hoopes, D. (1977). Effects of elevated plasma FFA and insulin on muscle glycogen usage during exercise. *Journal of Applied Physiology*, **43**, 695-699.

Costill, D.L., Sherman, W.M., Fink, W.J., Maresh, C., Witten, M., & Miller, J.M. (1981). The role of dietary carbohydrates in muscle glycogen resynthesis after strenuous running. *American Journal of Clinical Nutrition*, **34**, 1831-1836.

Coyle, E.F., Coggan, A.R., Hemmert, M.K., Lowe, R.C., & Walters, T.J. (1985). Substrate usage during exercise following a preexercise meal. *Journal of Applied Physiology*, **59**, 429-433.

Coyle, E.F., Hagberg, J.M., Hurley, B.F., Martin, W.H., Ehsani, A.A., & Holloszy, J.O. (1983). Carbohydrate feeding during prolonged strenuous exercise can delay fatigue. *Journal of Applied Physiology*, **55**, 230-235.

Davies, K.J.A., Maguire, J.J., Brooks, G.A., Dallman, P.R., & Packer, L. (1982). Muscle mitochondrial bioenergetics, oxygen supply, and work capacity during dietary iron deficiency and repletion. *American Journal of Physiology*, **242**, E417-E427.

Foster, C., Costill, D.L., & Fink, W.J. (1979). Effects of preexercise feeding on endurance performance. *Medicine and Science in Sports and Exercise*, **11**, 1-5.

Horstman, D., Weiskopf, R., & Jackson, R.E. (1980). Work capacity during 3-wk sojourn at 4,300 m: Effects of relative polycythemia. *Journal of Applied Physiology*, **49**, 311-318.

Ivy, J.L., Katz, S.L., Cutler, C.L., Sherman, W.M., & Coyle, E.F. (1988). Muscle glycogen synthesis after exercise: Effect of time of carbohydrate ingestion. *Journal of Applied Physiology*, **64**, 1480-1485.

Karlsson, J., & Saltin, B. (1971). Diet, muscle glycogen, and endurance performance. *Journal of Applied Physiology*, **31**, 203-206.

Neufer, P.D., Costill, D.L., Flynn, M.G., Kirwan, J.P., Mitchell, J.B., & Houmard, J. (1987). Improvements in exercise performance: Effects of carbohydrate feedings and diet. *Journal of Applied Physiology*, **62**, 983-988.

Nose, H., Mack, G.W., Shi, X., Morimoto, K., & Nadel, E.R. (1990). Effect of saline infusion during exercise on thermal and circulatory regulations. *Journal of Applied Physiology*, **69**, 609-616.

Powers, S.K., Lawler, J., Dodd, S., Tulley, R., Landry, G., & Wheeler, K. (1990). Fluid replacement drinks during high intensity exercise: Effects on minimizing exercise-induced disturbances in homeostasis. *European Journal of Applied Physiology*, **60**, 54-60.

Reynafarje, C., Lozano, R., & Valdivieso, J. (1959). The polycythemia of high altitudes: Iron metabolism and related aspects. *Blood*, **14**, 433-455.

Rowland, T.W., Deisroth, M.B., Green, G.M., & Kelleher, J.F. (1988). The effect of iron therapy on exercise capacity of nonanemic iron-deficient adolescent runners. *American Journal of Diseases in Children*, **142**, 165-169.

Sherman, W.M., Costill, D.L., Fink, W.J., & Miller, J.M. (1981). Effect of exercise-diet manipulation on muscle glycogen and its subsequent utilization during performance. *International Journal of Sports Medicine*, **2**, 114-118.

Sherman, W.M., & Wimer, G.S. (1991). Insufficient dietary carbohydrate during training: Does it impair athletic performance? *International Journal of Sport Nutrition*, **1**, 28-44.

Wilber, R.L. (1990). *Influence of glucose polymer ingestion on plasma glucose concentration and performance in male distance runners*. Unpublished master's thesis, Florida State University.

Williams, M.H., Wesseldine, S., Somma, T., & Schuster, R. (1981). The effect of induced erythrocythemia upon 5-mile treadmil run time. *Medicine and Science in Sports and Exercise*, **13**, 169-175.

Nagging Questions About the Pursuit of Excellence as a Justification for Enhancing Performance in Sport

R. Scott Kretchmar
Penn State University

Enhancing human performance would seem to be a fairly bland topic for a philosopher to address. If enhancing performance means improving it, and if the sorts of performances we have in mind are certain sport, dance, exercise, and other human movements that promote various goods while causing no appreciable harm, it would seem that this topic is not only bland but also philosophically uninteresting. In light of this, I could try to show that the concept of enhancing is more complicated than it appears to be, or that sport, dance, and exercise are not always as benign as they might seem. However, there is an alternative here that I think might bear more fruit.

I would like to spice up the topic of enhancing performance with the politically charged and philosophically complex issue of excellence. In addition, I want to examine one interpretation of what it is to be excellent in specifically human ways. I will look at both of these topics as justifications for enhancing performance, as reasons for wanting to get better at something and for working at it. In other words, were someone to ask, "Why is it that you would ever want to enhance performance?" I would like to be able to give the following as at least one possible answer: "I want to become humanly excellent." Or to put it more broadly and completely, "I want to become excellent in specifically human ways relative to the performance at hand."

Alasdair MacIntyre's notion of "practices" (1984, pp. 181-203) will serve here as a vehicle by which I will develop my ideas.[1] Many of you are aware of MacIntyre's analysis in his best-known book, *After Virtue*. You are probably also aware that this volume has been both celebrated and heavily criticized.[2] Some of these strengths and weaknesses will become evident in the course of my analysis, so I will not delay matters here to carry out a critique. However, I do need to review MacIntyre's project in order to establish the context for his important notion of practices.

The problem MacIntyre (1984) identifies is this: In our contemporary world we still have "isolated fragments" of an older morality (p. 2). Unfortunately, the original context that gave life and, more important, authority to these fragments, has long since vanished. Thus we are raised today in the company of such virtues as wisdom, courage, reason, and honesty, but we learn or sense that these values are not binding. Not only do we not agree on which values are "true" or which take precedence over others, we have lost our very ability to adjudicate rival value claims (pp. 6, 142-143).

Consequently we have a number of mostly vestigial virtues lying around, not doing the work they once did but still giving some of us vague feelings of guilt when we violate them. In short, what is left of virtues today does more to bother and confuse us than to enlighten and direct our actions.

For example, most of us would claim that cheating is wrong. Yet many of us may be ambivalent about the legitimacy of certain forms of rule bending or cheating. Can people who cheat at a game still be playing that game? Moreover, can they cheat and still win that game? Should they be honored if they build up fine records, in part, by cheating? Some say yes, others no, still others say "it depends." We are not sure what to do with the Jim Valvanos, Gaylord Perrys, Pete Roses, and Ben Johnsons of the sporting world. Give them prime time TV jobs? Put them in the Hall of Fame? Allow them to compete again after relatively short suspensions? Or banish them forever?

We are not sure what to make of intentional fouls in basketball. Are they simply strategy, or are they morally dubious acts? We are not sure what to make of intimidation in hockey, football, and even basketball. Should we praise it as a robust and courageous technique designed to promote a victory? Or should we condemn it as a form of cheating?

MacIntyre would say (though he does not address all of these sport related issues directly) that we no longer have any reasoned way to solve such problems. The weak presence of virtues may make us uneasy with cheating or drug taking or acts of intimidation, but our inability to convincingly argue our case leaves us at best ambivalent and stoic spectators, if not active participants, under our contemporary "live and let live" philosophy (pp. 169-170).

We put up with different definitions of success; we are patient with "evil" acts and "different" people. Because we no longer share common virtues in the world of sport, we lack community. We lack the warm fellowship gained from marching together toward common ends. We retreat to individualism and stoic endurance.

MacIntyre traces this problem to a cluster of related events. The root cause, MacIntyre claims, is the loss of an Aristotelian vision of humankind as having a character (essential nature) and proper function (essential end or telos) (pp. 52-55). Without a reliable sense of people as they could be if they realized their essential nature, there is no ground against which to measure people as they happen to be, and no rational grounding for the virtues which, of course, are designed to transport people from their "untutored state" to their true end. "Ethics therefore in this view presupposes some account of potentiality and act, some account of the essence of man as a rational animal and above all some account of the human *telos*" (p. 52).

Put in other terms, an inability or unwillingness to speculate on and describe human excellence created the is-to-ought problem. If, as science has claimed, we can only describe in value neutral terms what a person is, there may indeed be an unbridgable gap between is and ought. However, if we can describe a person in an ideal state, just as we seem to be able to distinguish excellent cars, newspapers, or baseball teams from poor ones, and just as we seem to be able to describe the specific qualities that make them fine examples of their species, then ought is implicit in the identification and description.

There is no logical problem. In seeing and describing human life, we are seeing and describing it in terms of its potential to be, in terms of its telos. MacIntyre thinks there is an in-built obligation to attempt to realize this end, for it would be illogical to claim both that this is what human beings are *at their best* and there is no need to attempt to achieve it.

According to MacIntyre then, with a teleological conception of human nature in hand, there is no logical problem of moving from is to ought. Rather we are moving from is to is, from fact to fact, from what the true nature of personhood is to what a person must do if he or she is to be true to this nature (p. 59).

But MacIntyre did not go through all this just to dwell on the failure of liberal individualism or to convince us that all of this is caused by our abandonment of some Aristotelian, teleological view of life. He presents a three-step antidote or cure for our moral ills, and this is where his notion of practices fits in. The adoption (or re-adoption) of practices is the first of three steps, all of which must be taken according to MacIntyre, if one is to construct a life that reflects human excellence.

Teleological Practice Ethics

A practice for MacIntyre is somewhat difficult to describe. He says that throwing a football is not a practice but that a game of football is (p. 187). Miscellaneous cooking is not a practice, but the art of baking is. MacIntyre defines a practice in terms of goods that can be realized. The game of football is a practice because it has any number of internal goods that can be achieved only by attempting to play football well. For example, creative running and beautiful fakes are goods that accrue to persons who dedicate themselves to being good football players. On the other hand, these goods do not necessarily come to those who pursue values that are extrinsic to the practice of football, say, to fame or even victory, for those can be achieved by cheating or through an official's bad call, luck, or any number of other means.

A virtue, then, is that which leads to or allows an individual to achieve goods that are internal to a practice. For example, an individual might need integrity in order to confront football's skill requirements head-on rather than to look for shortcuts, tricks, or other ways to cheat the game, if not also his opponents. Integrity would lead to a person's ability someday to display his skills of running, tackling, and blocking (i.e., various goods internal to football) and to be honored for them. In so doing, assuming he has some aptitude for the game, he will achieve some degree of excellence. If he is particularly gifted, he may even help to redefine what it is to be excellent at football.

In MacIntyre's own words, a practice is "a coherent and complex form of socially established cooperative human activity through which goods internal to that form of activity are realized in the course of trying to achieve those standards of excellence which are appropriate to, and partially definitive of, that form of activity, with the result that human powers to achieve excellence, and human conceptions of the ends and goods involved, are systematically extended'' (1984, p. 187).

MacIntyre, as noted earlier, supplements his recommendation that people engage in practices with two additional suggestions. The first is that people build their practices into a coherent narrative aimed at the good life. It is important that people become the authors of their lives, authors of a story that is leading somewhere. It is not enough to engage in practices in any willy-nilly, random, illegal, or harm-causing way. Rather, individuals should see themselves on a path that, in spite of its twists and turns, makes sense. It is always, if unevenly, about themselves and their quest for the good life.

This provides a second foundation for virtues. Integrity, for example, might be needed if a person is to claim and own various actions in his or her life, even those that turn out to be embarrassments or failures (Feldman, 1986, p. 309). All actions should be part of a person's unfolding story and bear the signature, if only faintly, of the author.

Content for the good life, according to MacIntyre, is supplied by tradition. The roles that people assume and the character of the ends that people ought to pursue are made intelligible from within a historical tradition. The virtues that sustain and extend practices consequently also sustain and extend traditions. Vices undermine practices in a culture and ultimately lead to the extinction of cultural identity through tradition.

Feldman (1986), Wartofsky (1984), Frankena (1983), Downing and Thigpen (1984), and others have pointed out numerous problems with this analysis ranging from the obvious (e.g., MacIntyre's inability to avoid ethical relativism, given his emphasis on historical traditions for determining the content of practices) to the more esoteric (e.g., ambiguities over the location of the telos; is it found in social roles or in the quest?) (Downing & Thigpen, 1984). Nevertheless, MacIntyre holds an elevated view both of humankind and of these things he calls practices. Both allow us to gain what I think is something of a new vision of sport and those who are engaged in it. Or perhaps, more in the spirit of MacIntyre's work itself, these help us regain portions of an older view of athletes and sport.

Four Steps in Pursuing Human Excellence

Here I will defend a secular form of teleology that avoids—as indeed MacIntyre himself wished to do—any form of Aristotelian biological teleology. In the process I will identify some of the requisite virtues that would be needed if individuals are to make such progress during their lifetime. I will also defend against two criticisms that would question the rational ground for ethical decision making within practices. My position is not without presupposition, but I hope it is plausible and provocative.

I believe that we humans take a step (perhaps a small one, but a step nevertheless) toward reaching our nature—what we are at our best—when we acknowledge the difference between internal and external ends.[3] This is a feat of reason and, as far as I know, an accomplishment that is within the grasp only of specifically human levels of intelligence.

External ends, as noted before, are things like fame, money, and possibly even victories in sport. These are external because they can be described independently of any specified means, that is, they are intelligible apart from any necessary means. As we know, fame and wealth can be gained in any number of different ways, both legal and illegal, both noble and ignoble. Even victories can be gained through skill, or luck, or an official's bad call. They can be secured through playing by the rules or by cheating.

Internal goods are those sorts of things that are inseparable from certain means. One cannot show excellence in football, for example, without confronting football's problems head-on and dealing with them honestly. One cannot be a fine modern dancer without confronting the issues of creative expression courageously and directly. One cannot have the best curveball in baseball without using the same allowable means available to other pitchers who aspire to throwing the best curveball.

MacIntyre argues, and I agree, that if one cheats in chess one cannot be an excellent chess player (given the nature of the chess problem as defined by its constitutive rules), even though one could conceivably win in a technical sense and even become rich and famous if one's cheating were not discovered or if no one cared that the cheating had occurred.

Once this distinction has been made, we need to take the second step—that being to make a value judgment on which type of good, internal or external, is of greater significance. Internal goods, it would seem, deserve the higher ranking because they are the sorts of things that are experienced as satisfactory in their own right. That is, they are ends in themselves; they are excellences. The experiences of beautiful diving, creative shot-making, shrewd defensive reacting, graceful stroking, peaceful anticipating, unusually high leaping into the air, and countless other sport excellences are intrinsically good. Again, they are good in themselves; we do not feel obligated to explain what they are good for.

On the other hand, external goods such as fame and fortune may be experienced as intrinsically good, but they are frequently used merely as means to other experiences that are good in their own right. The intrinsic power of these goods is also often short-lived, perhaps because their inherent properties are weak, or perhaps because (as external goods) we may be able to take no credit for having won them. We can become rich and famous because of family ties, quite apart from any effort or the display of any excellence on our part. In any case, the closer ties of internal goods to intrinsic value would give us a reason to judge those goods as superior, as the ones that we ought to pursue most vigorously.

A third step in the movement toward human excellence comes then in the identification and development of those means that give one access to various internal goods. As argued above, such means necessarily require the exhibition of virtues. MacIntyre singles out honesty, justice, and courage as three virtues essential to involvement in practices. A virtue, he says, "*is an aquired human quality, the possession and exercise of which tends to enable us to achieve those goods which are internal to practices and the lack of which effectively prevents us from achieving any such goods*" (p. 191).

A fourth step in the pursuit of human life in its highest form is taken when we recognize and celebrate the achievement of internal goods, particularly in the direction of excellence. I say direction because I do not believe there is any one ideal, terminal state of affairs in any sport that must be reserved for the term excellence. Nor is excellence something that requires a zero-sum model. The fact that you have just defeated me in a 100-meter dash does not preclude the possibility that *both* of us displayed excellence in that race. If a good portion of the world's population dedicated themselves to the practice of golf, there is every reason to believe that most of them would achieve a high level of excellence.[4]

All this is consistent with MacIntyre's position. However, I part company with him when he argues that excellence must be historically understood (p. 189). I think there are objective standards for excellence, even though these essential benchmarks are always embellished and often complemented with culture-relative appreciations. For example, in a dash, faster is better, and this is not at all a matter of the historical development of running or of culture-specific variables. While some cultures and time periods may prefer graceful running to running with power, or lightening starts to steady starts and fast finishes, or running ahead rather than coming from behind, excellence in the dash still objectively and necessarily lies in the direction of faster rather than slower.[5]

In any case, it is an important step in the pursuit of human excellence to mark such successes, to notice when they happen, and to appreciate such gains. The fine display of skill, cunning, artistry, or perception that is required by a given practice may not occur as regularly as one would like. At the highest levels it is a genuinely special event. But at various stages in the quest for what might be called practice mastery, noticing and celebrating the successive acquisition of internal goods is properly human and humanly important.

This may, paradoxically, fall at odds with the realization of various external ends. But again humans, in contrast to lower forms of animal life, can acknowledge this difference. Even though a game might be lost, excellence might be achieved. The display of skill is acknowledged and appreciated for its own sake.

The second aspect of success, according to MacIntyre (1984, pp. 188-189), is the appreciation received from those who are members of the practice family. This appreciation receives its significance from its source. It comes from those who "have been there," who are members of the club, who know what they are seeing, who can appreciate the intricacies of skill and strategy. These are people who have also dedicated themselves to the practice at hand. Thus, while the loudest noises may come from fans who are not members of the guild and who therefore may focus on various irrelevancies, the most significant reactions will come from brother or sister artists who may, after a performance, walk over and simply whisper, "That was good."

It is now clear why practices are a corrective for liberal idealism. Practices generate family and friendship. Those who stand in relationship to a practice, whether it be painting, potting, or basketball, stand in subordination to *it*. *It* holds them together; *it* is what attracts their attention; *it* is what seems to provide never-ending challenges and fascination. The practice stands between people and gives them a common focus. Because virtues are required to participate in a practice, it also gives them a common ethic.

To summarize, part of what it is to be human is to see the differences between internal and external ends, acknowledge the superiority of internal ends, develop the virtues that are needed in order to pursue and achieve such ends, and acknowledge and celebrate such achievements when they occur. Animals know nothing of the difference between playing and playing well, between winning and winning well. Because they are not rational in this sense, they would have no basis upon which to develop virtues. While animals might pursue prey playfully or desperately, they cannot pursue it honestly, justly, or courageously. Animals, in short, cannot become connoisseurs of fine movement, outstanding skill, and superior cunning even though in certain ways they can display these achievements.[6]

Two Potential Difficulties With a Teleological Practice Ethics

There are at least two questions that may appear to have no answer on the basis of this MacIntyre-inspired notion of human excellence. First, what if two individuals have conflicting beliefs regarding the scope or definition of a practice? On the basis of reason, how is such a conflict to be resolved? And second, what if two apparent virtues in a practice require a person to do two different things? Again, on the basis of reason, how is a person to decide which virtue takes precedence?

Many cases of conflict regarding the scope or limits of a practice have to do with new technique and technology. For a number of years in top-level table tennis, for instance, it has been common practice for some players to put very different types of rubber on the two sides of their paddle or bat. One sheet of rubber is tacky and thus graps the ball and imparts a tremendous spin determined by bat angle and the direction of the arm swing. On the other side of the paddle, players put a rubber that has precisely the opposite effect. This surface allows the ball to skid and retain its original spin even though bat angle and the direction of the arm swing make it look otherwise to an opponent.

When these rubber sheets were first manufactured and some players became accomplished at using this new technology, some expressed a concern that this would ruin the game. Certain spins, it was thought, would be undetectible, and certian shots would be virtually unreturnable. But as so often happens in sport, after some time the defense eventually caught up with the offense. Ironically, most of those who feared this new technology and thought it would ruin table tennis came to realize that it actually made the game more complex and interesting. There was more to learn; there was both better defense and a more varied offense to master. In short there were increasingly diverse ways to play excellently in a game that retained a good balance between new ways to make problems and solve them.

Nevertheless, no one was prepared for what happened next: A few Eastern players developed the technique of spinning their rackets below the top of the table between shots so that the rubber that was on the forehand side might be different on any two successive forehand shots. They used the same color of rubber for both sides of the bat so the opponent would have no clue as to the type of rubber (spin reversing or preserving) being used. Interestingly and relevantly, this technique was legal.

Now the dilemma: Were not the players who developed and used this technique to be praised and honored for their efficiency in legally deceiving their opponents? In fact they produced deception far more efficiently and effectively than anyone had ever done before. What would keep them from saying, in effect, that now there is a new practice of table tennis and that they are to be the most honored among the new family members? Who is to say what table tennis is today or what it is to be tomorrow? Who is to say that this skill is or is not to stand as an arena of internal excellence for table tennis?

I think that MacIntyre would have an answer, or if he does not, I will supply him with one. This brand of efficiency, this technique for enhancing performance, even though it was legal, turned out to diminish the craft, art, or practice of table tennis. This is not merely an aesthetic opinion. It is based in a motor perceptual fact. Simply, the balls hit with this novel technique cannot be returned. Or better said, opponents are reduced to guessing which side of the paddle had in fact contacted the ball. If they guess right, they might be successful in returning the shot. If they guess wrong, the ball has no chance of striking the table. The defensive side of the game, under this practice, is turned into a 50–50 game of roulette.

And that dramatically impoverishes the activity! It simplifies the problem in the sense of making it boring; it reduces the significance of skill in playing the game; it replaces creative responses, in part, with the table tennis equivalent of flipping a coin. And moreover, those in the table tennis family, those who know best, say there is no realistic possibility for a defensive adjustment as there was with the earlier innovation that initially gave the advantage to the offense.

Is there a reason then, some objective ground, for determining which new efficiencies, which game evolutions, are advances for a practice and which are not? There is, but it is not to be found among the virtues. The issue cannot be solved by encouraging these players to be honest, courageous, and just. On some criteria they were these things. They followed the rules and were well within their legal rights. But it can, I think, be solved by examining the character of the practice in question here, namely the game of table tennis.

This is not a matter of looking for any unchangeable essence of table tennis. But it is one of searching for the preservation or improvement of the test that is provided by the convention called table tennis. This is a practical problem of determining what makes for a richer, more interesting, complex, and riveting test. In the case of long-standing, successful practices like table tennis, we begin this analysis in a position of subordination to the game, with a degree of respect for it.

The judgment of generations has been that table tennis, prior to the paddle spinning technique, was indeed rich, interesting, complex, and riveting. The judgment of generations has been that there is a marvelous and possibly inexhaustible kingdom there. It takes patience, sacrifice, and determination to participate partly or more fully in its goods. A degree of subordination to the historical practice and reverence for its qualities is appropriate, even required.

Yet this subordination and reverence should never be absolute. Table tennis has no essential, unchanging nature; it has no ideal form that it ''strives'' to achieve; it was not ordained by God or anyone else to be forever one way and not another. Practices are evolving conventions, forever in need of improvement, never reaching any final or ideal form. But from this it does not follow that practice evolution is the product of whim, taste, or personal opinion.

Nor does it follow then that virtues are relative to whatever one thinks or fancies that a practice should be. Or to put it another way, honesty in confronting a game's problems cannot be reduced to a legalistic requirement that players merely follow the rules. Plumbing the deep riches of internal excellences available in this activity, MacIntyre might say, is more successful when the virtue of honesty is understood to entail more than simple rule adherence.

Consequently, there would appear to be reason-based decisions here relative to the ways in which the practice of table tennis should and should not be allowed to evolve. The use of various new sheets of rubber should be permitted, and the technique of spinning the table tennis racket under the table should be prohibited.[7] The supposedly irreconcilable conflict between different forms of a practice is found to be rationally reconcilable after all.[8] Furthermore, the virtue of honesty is found to require more than adherence to only the letter of the law. When a new technique, even a legal one, harms the very practice that gave rise to it, honesty urges players not to use it.

A second potential difficulty with this teleological, practice-based ethic is raised by Susan Feldman (1986). She argues that MacIntyre does not successfully avoid relativism because, within practices themselves, there are conflicting virtues that have equal legitimacy. She refers to an ambiguous shot in tennis. Honestly uncertain as to whether the ball hit by her opponent landed in or out, what should she do? Should she call the shot "in" or "out"? Here is a portion of her analysis:

> My call could go either way, without being clearly wrong. If I am a particularly competitive player, and surely competitiveness is a virtue in playing games, then I will be inclined to give myself the advantage. If I have the trait of "good sportsmanship" more strongly than competitiveness, then I will be inclined to give the advantage to my opponent. Thus, in ambiguous cases, tennis related virtues themselves lead to different judgments.

> To insist that one call is right, and the other wrong, is to assume that one tennis related virtue is more important than another. But it is not clear just how one can weigh virtues. Each trait focuses on a different vision of the good gained by games, and different conceptions of excellence in tennis (winning vs. being a good sport). There is no non-arbitrary way to settle this dispute. (p. 311)

On the contrary, I think that the framework provided by MacIntyre does indeed give us a nonarbitrary way to settle this dispute, though the settlement in this case is a bit unusual if not amusing. Feldman has misconstrued the nature of tennis and consequently provided a misleading description of the dilemma. It is misleading in a way that gives her the conclusion she wants.

The critical issue in practices, as noted above, is the preservation and enhancement of the opportunities to gain and experience the various goods internal to that practice. Whatever behavior is chosen, it should be consistent with that end. But Feldman believes she has hold of two contradictory behaviors, based on two virtues. She sees it as a matter of taste or opinion as to whether sportsmanship (giving the point away) or competitiveness (taking the point) should prevail.

However, do either of these decisions affect the participants' capacity to achieve various goods that are internal to the practice of tennis? If tennis and its goods necessarily involve the solution of temporal/spatial problems involving moving balls, rackets, numbers of bounces, nets, and a specified court, then it would seem that either decision would be equally good. If I am honestly uncertain about where the shot landed, my calling it "in" does nothing to diminish opportunities for solving such problems. Nor, as a matter of fact, does my calling it "out." The integrity of the game is not threatened or affected whatsoever with either call. It is only the fallibility of my eyesight, not my moral reasoning, that forces on me this dilemma of conflicting virtues and requires the begrudging necessity to guess at a call.

To put it another way, the internal goods of tennis are not related to magnanimity (giving away a point that I might in fact have earned—what Feldman, curiously, calls sportsmanship). Nor is it related to selfishness (taking a point that I might in fact not deserve—what Feldman, curiously, calls competitiveness). It is possible of course to have a craft or practice develop around various sensitivities and skills of magnanimity or selfishness, but it is difficult to see what they have to do directly or necessarily with the practice of tennis.

What is crucial to the practice of tennis is getting the call right, for without right calls both the tennis problems and the skills and artistry needed to solve them are diminished or otherwise threatened. But in this particular case no one knows what the right call is. Consequently, my opponent and I could play entirely ethical matches in any of the following ways regarding the dilemma in question. We could agree that each person will call any undiscernible ball, for which it is his or her responsibility to make the call, in his or her own favor. Or to put a more generous face on this, we could call each such shot in favor of our opponent. Or, on the chance that such an agreement might create an injustice, each party could agree to alternate judgments on ambiguous balls, the first one in your favor, the second in mine, and so on throughout the match. Of course it is also possible in unofficial matches to play undiscernible balls over.

Feldman, in effect, has identified a pseudoproblem for MacIntyre's system. Ironically, calling a ball "in" or "out" is virtue and ethics neutral in this case. Neither call affects the integrity of the practice of tennis or its internal goods. Neither call is grounded in a competing virtue of tennis.

Good sportsmanship, under MacIntyre's view, would be expressed in a concern that "calls are gotten right," not in a feeling that the points I might have deserved but am not sure about should be given automatically to my opponent. And the virtue of competitiveness would be expressed in a concern to do my best to outdistance my opponent in a situation in which the calls are gotten right, not in a feeling that the points I might not deserve should be given automatically to me. But again, because no one knows which call is right, an agreement or convention is needed here to keep the game moving and to minimize the potential for injustice to either party.

Some might object that I have dismissed these potential dilemmas too easily. Is it not possible that an individual could reject the whole notion of internal goods or internal excellences? What forces anyone, in other words, to agree that involvement in practices is at least one key element in the good life? Why couldn't a person take a stand on external goods, on success, on the cultivation of efficiency for securing desirable objects or states of affairs quite apart from any concern with skill, cunning, artistry, creativity, and the virtues that allow such internal goods to become available?

The answer, at least for MacIntyre, refers us back to his claim about our ability to see and describe human life in its good forms. MacIntyre, I think, would argue that we are not rationally free to adopt this form of life because it is inconsistent with humankind at its best. It would be to live a life in which one acknowledges knowing what one ought to be but chooses to act as one ought not to be.

Can we tell a good table from a bad one? Granted that it is more difficult to tell a good human from a bad one, is it still impossible in principle to do so? MacIntyre thinks not, and I agree. I have argued that we possess certain capabilities that distinguish and elevate us, if they are exercised and developed. I claimed that some of these have to do with recognitions of internal and external ends and of the necessary relationship between certain means and internal ends in practices. I argued that some of these have to do with judgments regarding of the superior value of internal goods or excellences in contrast to external ends. I suggested that a practice ethic has a rational foundation that permits the resolution of different competing conceptions of practices and the competing authority found in two virtues.

Implications of a Practice Based Ethic for Physical Education

This emphasis on a teleological conception of humankind and an involvement in practices has some interesting implications for our field generally, and the topic of enhancing human performance in particular. I would like to end by listing several deductions that strike me as reasonably significant.

1. It is far more useful to examine excellences that are *peculiar to and embedded in* practices than it is to deal with performance success in the abstract. Citius, altius, fortius (faster, higher, stronger) is obviously relevant to practice excellence in sport, but on its own it is unhelpfully generic, abstract, cold, and clinical. The promise of excellence, then, needs to be tied to one or more specific crafts, to the virtues that allow one to achieve the goods that are internal to those crafts, and to the hope that someday the community, after observing one's performance, will say, "That was good." Consequently, we should seek to enhance performance, not simply to allow our students, athletes, and movement clients to reach some mechanically defined and mathematically measured state of perfection but rather to join fraternities and sororities of people who relish the quest and satisfactions involved in playing well.

2. Wellsprings for human excellence are encountered in local, idiosyncratic, and evolving cultural games, dances, and exercises. This has implications for how we conceive of ourselves, even what we call ourselves. If we understand that human excellence does not necessarily lie in the direction of the abstract in contrast to the particular, or in the more universal rather than the local, then there is little reason to flee from or apologize for our curious games, dances, and other cultural practices. If we go further than this to agree that excellence requires a commitment to one or more specific practices, then we might even want to focus on the particular more than on the abstract—on baseball, horseshoes, and Hungarian folk dances rather than movement, mechanical models of objects moving through space, and stroke volumes.

3. This understanding, however, does not place baseball above science, or horseshoes closer to human excellence than kinesiology. Science too can be engaged in as a practice with its own set of internal excellences. Consequently, science and sport, kinesiology and dance, biomechanics and exercise are, in principle, on a par with one another. Just as there are fraternities of clay scientists and sororities of potters, there are and should be guilds of movement scientists and associations of table tennis artists.

4. Sport and other cultural movement forms, considered as practices, have close affinities with art. Sport has, in part, the structure and character of art. Sport presents a dilemma, the resolution of which presents any number of opportunities for the display of creativity, insight, inventiveness, and many other excellences. So too with aesthetic, pedagogical, academic, medical, and any number of other significant problematics around which a practice can form. A painter, for example, faces problems related to color, space, shape, and texture in the attempt to convey an idea or impression. Also, one of the very important excellences of sport is shared by art itself—that of aesthetic beauty or goodness. While different sports vary in the degree to which they tap into this source of excellence, all sports pay it homage by acknowledging that, all else being equal, a graceful and successful move is superior to one that is only successful.

5. Sport, in its most powerful form, has close affinities with play. It is a fascination with the various excellences of one's peculiar practice that sustain continued involvement. If fascination assures autotelicity (the lived acknowledgment that the doing or questing is its own reward), then much of the time spent in practices is spent in the stance or spirit of play. Empirically, it is difficult to understand how we would become accomplished at our practice unless we mostly loved it, unless we were at least partly at *its* beck and call. And philosophically, it is difficult to understand why we would become devotees to a practice unless we found ''something of meaning'' there. For both reasons, and probably others, play has much to do with the value of our field and the human successes of each one of us individually.

6. MacIntyre has not generated ideas that have not already, at least in part, been pursued in our exercise and sport science literature. Here are a few of the writers who, I believe, have shed considerable light on the significance of sport, dance, and exercise in ways that anticipated or at least are consistent with MacIntyre. Johan Huizinga (1950) saw that play both supported the development of human culture and that it did so in a variety of places—on the job, at leisure, in politics, in art, and in sport. (MacIntyre, I think, would endorse play as the mode in which practices best flourish. I think he would also applaud the absence of intellectual elitism, evident in Huizinga's work, regarding where play or practices may be found and where it is that culture is developed.)

Eleanor Metheny (1968) at once sensed a relationship between sport and art and saw the relative unimportance of the distinction between verbal and nonverbal thinking and expression. (MacIntyre, I think, would be impressed with her insight about the equivalence of meaning in sport and art and her high valuation of what we might call the nonverbal practices.) Michael Novak (1976) argued for the importance of differences between diverse kinds of practices—between football, basketball, and baseball—and also saw sport at its finest in the mode of play rather than work. (MacIntyre would probably applaud his emphasis on the distinctions between different sports or practices and the kinds of excellences that are found in each. He would also undoubtedly support his emphasis on sport in the spirit of play.)

Michael Polanyi (1966; Polanyi & Prosch, 1975) provided important analyses of the fundamental similarities of all arts (including the movement arts) and of the human superiority of art over other sorts of activities. (MacIntyre, I believe, would concur that inventiveness and creativity, wherever they are found, are excellences or internal goods of practices.) Bernard Suits (1978) saw games as a particularly significant form of human involvement and argued consistently that no apologies need be given for the time devoted to them. (MacIntyre, interestingly, uses games as an exemplar of what he has in mind when he speaks of practices. One never has the sense, when reading MacIntyre, that a game is merely a game.)

Finally, David Sudnow (1978) traced his virtue-supported quest for the internal excellencies available in jazz piano. (MacIntyre, I speculate, would hold up Sudnow as a prototype of the virtuous individual, as one who is given honestly, courageously, and justly to the practice of jazz piano.)

Consequently, it is not so much that MacIntyre has produced an understanding of human excellence that has not occurred to anyone else. It is more that he has articulated, through his teleological understanding of humankind and his notion of practices, parts of what many different philosophers have seen before, if only dimly or from a slightly different angle.

There is no cheating rhetoric, philosophy, jazz piano, or football because such cheating requires less insight, good judgment, and dedication than we as humans are capable of. If we are to live the good life, a certain portion of our time and energy should be devoted to practices, whether in academe, sport, the fine arts, public service, various hobbies, or other endeavors. When we propose to enhance human performance, we would do well to present improvement in a game, dance, sport, exercise, or movement skill as one step in a respectful and ongoing involvement with a practice.

Taking some cues from MacIntyre's work, I have argued that virtue-grounded involvement in such a loving quest is itself a form of human excellence. The subsequent achievement of various levels of excellence internal to our practices (higher, faster, stronger, more beautiful. . .) then becomes a bonus. In such a world, my own nagging questions about the pursuit of excellence as a justification for enhancing performance in sport are largely laid to rest.

Notes

[1] I realize there is some danger in separating the concept of practices from those of narrative lifecourse and tradition. MacIntyre saw these as three interrelated and necessary aspects of his new rational ethics. My emphasis on practices, in effect, leaves unanswered important questions that prompted MacIntyre to speak of lifecourse coherence and the importance of historical traditions. I will attempt to acknowledge some of those questions at appropriate places in this essay but will have no opportunity to address them in any adequate way.

[2] See Downing and Thigpen (1984), Feldman (1986), Frankena (1983), and Wartofsky (1984).

[3] For a thorough discussion of different kinds of ends that are available in sport, see Fraleigh (1983). MacIntyre's notion of internal excellencies is broader than Fraleigh's description of the intrinsic value of sport from the moral point of view. Nevertheless, Fraleigh's interest in grounding sport in one or more inherent values is, I believe, entirely consistent with MacIntyre's understanding of internal goods.

[4] Of course it is not enough simply to give oneself to a practice. There is always the matter of aptitude for the practice in question and the possibility that individuals would not be able to display high levels of excellence in that particular activity no matter what

their degree of dedication and no matter how long they practiced. However, it seems clear that most individuals have sufficient psychomotor wherewithal to achieve at least modest threshold levels of excellence that would be specific to each activity and would show a "tension" between objective and subjective criteria.

[5]It could be claimed that I have selected an example favorable to my own objectivistic tendencies. Racing is an activity in which speed is unequivocally the desired quality. But what about baseball, football, or basketball, where tensions between power and speed, or grace and cunning, seem historically or culturally fluid? Here I would concede that games need not honor single qualities or even require that various qualities or features of skillful play fall in any set order. Nevertheless, after having admitted to a certain openness with regard to the character of excellence displayed in various games, I would also argue that this openness has objective limits.

[6]This position is not a revisitation of the old moralism captured by Grantland Rice's well-known saying, "When the One Great Scorer comes to write against your name—He marks—not that you won or lost—but how you played the game" (Bartlett, 1980, p. 773). Neither does it stand in clear support of those who would argue that sport teaches character. Sport is not a stage on which one displays moral ideals apart from winning or losing, apart from playing skillfully or not. Sport is a craft, the whole point of which is to provide an opportunity for the development and display of skill, insight, creativity, and other manifestations of excellence.

[7]Within some limits, governing bodies have permitted the use of a remarkable variety of smooth and dimpled rubber sheets. On the other hand, the International Table Tennis Federation modified game rules to neutralize the game-damaging technique of flipping the bat below the level of the table. Players who hit with both sides of their bat must now cover each with different colored rubber. Consequently, opponents know which side of the bat was used on each shot by the person at the other end of the table. By this action, the guessing element is reduced or eliminated and the skill element is restored.

[8]This is not to say that all decisions will be easy, but only that the grounds for making decisions will be clear and unavoidable. In some ways my cases were relatively easy ones with which to deal. The new rubber sheets improved possibilities for skillful and creative shotmaking. The new racket spinning technique, conversely, had rather clear negative effects on the game. In other cases, however, even experts might disagree on short-range and long-term effects of a new technique, an equipment change, or some constitutive rule modification.

References

Bartlett, J. (1980). *Familiar quotations*. Boston: Little & Brown.

Downing, L., & Thigpen, R. (1984). After *telos*: The implications of MacIntyre's attempt to restore the concept in *After Virtue*. *Social Theory and Practice*, **10**, 39-54.

Feldman, S. (1986). Objectivity, pluralism and relativism: Critique of MacIntyre's theory of virtue. *The Sourthern Journal of Philosophy*, **24**, 307-319.

Fraleigh, W. (1983). An examination of relationships of inherent, intrinsic, instrumental, and contributive values in the good sports contest. *Journal of the Philosophy of Sport*, **10**, 52-60.

Frankena, W. (1983). MacIntyre and modern morality. *Ethics*, **93**, 579-587.

Huizinga, J. (1950). *Homo ludens: A study of the play element in culture*. Boston: Beacon Press.

MacIntyre, A. (1984). *After virtue: A study in moral theory* (2nd ed.). Notre Dame, IN: University of Notre Dame Press.

Metheny, E. (1968). *Movement and meaning.* New York: McGraw Hill.

Novak, M. (1976). *The joy of sports: End zones, bases, baskets, balls, and the consecration of the American spirit.* New York: Basic Books.

Polanyi, M. (1966). *The tacit dimension.* New York: Doubleday.

Polanyi, M., & Prosch, H. (1975). *Meaning.* Chicago: University of Chicago Press.

Sudnow, D. (1978). *Ways of the hand: The organization of improvised conduct.* Cambridge, MA: Harvard University Press.

Suits, B. (1978). *The grasshopper: Games, life and utopia.* Toronto: University of Toronto Press.

Wartofsky, M. (1984). Virtue lost or understanding MacIntyre. *Inquiry, 27*, 235-250.

Enhancing Performance and Excellence in Sport—Some Critical Questions

Warren P. Fraleigh
SUNY, College at Brockport

Scott Kretchmar has given us a provocative and complex paper. It is the kind of paper that is difficult to react to because it has so much that requests attention. First, he indicates that enhancing performance itself is not a sufficient, or at least not the most important, reason for efforts to enhance performance. Something else, a stated rationale for why it is important for someone to become better, is needed.

He indicates also that the pursuit of excellence has been a siren call. We have all heard any number of justifications for enhancing performance in the pursuit of excellence. For example, NCAA Division I universities often cite pursuit of excellence as a justification for overfunded, overemphasized, and overvalued intercollegiate athletic programs. Frequently the *content* of excellence goes unspecified. Is it economic excellence? Or political excellence? Or educational excellence? Or human excellence? It is this latter that Kretchmar chooses as appropriate.

Let me now state what I want to talk about in this reaction. First, I want to distinguish between an ethics of virtue and an ethics of duty. That distinction can be crucial in determining how we choose the appropriate ethical efforts for enhancing human performance in sport. Second, I want to review several of the major points made by Kretchmar and to identify what significant but unanswered questions these points raise. Also, I will try to indicate why these questions are important to answer. And, finally, I want to identify a major difference I have with Scott's analysis, although this difference depends upon an assumption I make about what he intends.

Scott Kretchmar, and his source, Alisdair MacIntyre, have proposed an ethic of virtue. This type of ethic needs to be contrasted with an ethic of duty. Such a contrast will accomplish two things: It will clarify the kind of ethic proposed, and it will set the stage for a statement later about what these two kinds of ethics mean for the process of moral education.

An ethic of virtue is an ethic that depends on the character of persons for ethically correct action to take place. It may be called an ethic of ''being'' wherein a person acts in ethically right ways because he or she is a certain kind of person. For example, an honest person does honest things, is truthful, and so on. Furthermore, a person's character is not simply something he or she puts on like a coat;

figuratively, it is in his or her "biochemistry." Also, an honest person will do honest things because it is his or her character to do so; it comes naturally and does not require a careful calculation. Finally, an ethic of virtue means that the character traits, the virtues, are acquired, they are not wholly innate. So we may now see that in a general way the process of moral education is largely inculcating the virtues into people, that is, developing character.

In contrast, an ethic of duty depends upon the development of moral principles, maxims, or guides. Here the person refers his or her judgment to a rationally derived system of principles, maxims, or guides. These principles are brought to moral situations or issues to help the person decide on what the morally right action is. Accordingly, what the person does as the right action becomes a matter of *decision* using the relevant principles, and so forth, in the given situation or issue.

Some examples of the kinds of principles that inform an ethic of duty are Kant's categorical imperative which in one formulation says, "Treat other persons always as ends and never merely as means." Or, the principle of nonmaleficence which states that it is morally wrong to harm other persons intentionally and unnecessarily. Accordingly, the strategy for moral education with an ethic of duty is to instruct persons in the appropriate principles, the reasons in support of them, and to provide guided experiences in thinking through moral situations and issues using those principles.

As a summary contrast of these two types of ethics, we can see that an ethic of virtue would ask someone to be a benevolent, kind person while an ethic of duty would ask someone to act in accord with the principle of beneficence. A virtue ethic would ask someone to be fair while a duty ethic would ask someone to apply a principle of justice. A virtue ethic would ask us to be honest while a duty ethic would ask us to use a principle of veracity.

Now, I want to identify several points that are of major importance in Scott's paper and to raise some important questions from these points. First, he states that what is interesting philosophically in the topic of enhancing sports performance is what is an appropriate justification for doing so. Here he states that he wants to connect the idea of enhancing performance to that of excellence, but not a totally nondefined concept of excellence. By making this connection, he opens the way for putting content into excellence.

He rejects, implicitly, some possible ideas of excellence such as enhancing performance in order to secure more victories in the Olympics, a kind of political excellence. Or, he rejects enhancing performance for the sake of securing prizes or a high salary, a kind of economic excellence. He offers the justification for enhancing performance as a means of becoming "excellent in specifically human ways relative to the performance at hand," in this case sport.

So, from this we know that the content of the idea of excellence is to be that which is internal to the practice of sport. We also know that the excellence internal to the practice of sport is to be a terminal value, that is, a valued excellence that is intrinsically good and is not pursued, at least consciously, for the sake of such external excellences as political superiority or the highest salary in major league baseball.

To this point, Scott helps us look beyond the obvious and the mundane to justify enhancing performance. But there is a nagging question raised by

Kretchmar's analysis: What is specifically human excellence in the performance of sport? Paul Weiss, for instance, speaks of bodily excellence while Michael Novak discusses a kind of spiritual excellence. This question is dealt with only in obscure ways, and it begs for more complete discussion if we are to understand why this justification for enhancing performance is to be accepted as superior to many other possibilities.

A second major point of Kretchmar's is that a lack of common virtues in sport leaves us without a foundation upon which we can reach shared conclusions on what actions, motives, and intentions are morally acceptable. Thus we have become susceptible to an individualism that encourages a person to arrive at ethical judgments without reference to a tradition within which the individual is responsible for attaining and maintaining the commonweal. The question here is, How is it possible to arrive at common moral understanding if the individual is viewed as separate and distinct from a sustaining tradition? This question seems appropriate for the entire culture; it certainly is not restricted to sport.

Next, Scott discusses MacIntyre's position that a teleological conception of human nature can be the basis to which we refer questions of how we ought to be ethically. Such a foundation can provide common ends for humans, and because of such common ends, a practical ethic; that is, a common set of virtues can be imparted in accord with which the common ends become more achievable.

This point raises two significant questions: What is the ultimate telos of being human? And what is the compatible telos of being human in sport? If such questions are answered acceptably, then it is a relatively easy task to identify those virtues that are requisite. Answering such questions acceptably is a major difficulty. Buddhists have an answer, Christians have an answer, and rational humanists have an answer, but the substance of the answers is different. That leads to the problem of determining which is the "correct" answer or of locating a new and different answer that is correct. And what process or method will do so if modern philosophy has so far failed?

Using these bases from MacIntyre, Scott then outlines a three-factored teleological practice ethic. This ethic is to be applicable to the collective practice of sport, I presume, and to each particular sport individually. Here I will review the three elements in this outlined ethic and, once more, identify the questions that require attention.

The first element in the ethic is the distinction between the internal and external ends of sport and, importantly, the superior value of the internal ends over the external in becoming "excellent in specifically human ways relative to the performance at hand," sport. The question I see here is, What *are* these superior ends common to the sport practice and what are the corresponding internal ends unique to each sport? If we are to accept the pursuit of excellence in the internal goods of the sport practice as the important justification for enhancing performance, then we need clarity on what they are. Clarity on the ends to be pursued justifiably then provides guidance for the priority ends for biomechanists, physiologists, sport psychologists, and teachers and coaches in their efforts to enhance performance.

The second element in Kretchmar's practice ethic appears in two statements. First, "identification and development of those means that give one access to various internal goods" and "such means necessarily require the exhibition of virtues." There are two related questions to be asked here: What are these means that give access to the internal goods of sport? And how is it that the virtues of honesty, justice, and courage are required by these means? Answers to these questions together provide practical guidance for those who assist in enhancing performance as to what aspects of performance are important to improve (because they achieve the internal goods) and *how* such means are bettered in honest, just, and courageous ways.

The third element in Scott's practice ethic is recognizing and celebrating the achievement of internal goods. The question generated here is, What are the appropriate ways of recognizing the achievement of internal goods? This is significant. For as MacIntyre says, and Kretchmar reiterates, the institutions that sustain practices are very good at providing and promoting external goods such as fame, power, and material goods. In sport, the related institutions such as governing bodies, Olympic committees, the NCAA, and its constituent universities have become expert in emphasizing such external goods. They are so proficient at doing so that they divert sports practitioners from the internal goods and thus diminish the importance and priority of the internal goods and their accompanying virtues.

This negative impact of the institutions of sport upon the proper priority of the internal goods of sport brings me to one more overarching question suggested by Scott's paper. Indeed, this question would address the varied perspectives on improving sports performance included in this Academy program: What are the major constraints upon the ethically appropriate means of enhancing sports performance physiologically, psychologically, biomechanically, and pedagogically? This is a question for fruitful interaction between competent ethicists and those agents who attempt to enhance performance from these different perspectives.

In the spirit of exploration, and recognizing that I certainly have not had the time to pursue extended scholarship on this question, let me give some tentative, general answers to the question. For one illustration, acceptable physiological and biomechanical means of enhancing performance must be constrained by a standard of safety for athletes, for opponents, for all involved. Psychological means of performance enhancement must contribute positively to and not detract from viewing fellow competitors as facilitators in the mutual quest for human excellence in sports performance. Improving performance by means of teaching and coaching must focus on valuing the achievement of the internal goods of sport and relegating external and contradictory goods to secondary importance.

Now, how can those agents who enhance performance exhibit the important virtues championed by MacIntyre and seconded by Kretchmar? Again, in exploratory and simplistic fashion, let me provide outlines for how such agents may exhibit the virtues of justice, honesty, and courage.

First, they can enhance performance justly by openly sharing those successful means of doing so rather than restricting access to selected individuals, teams, or nations. Second, they can enhance performance honestly by recognizing publicly when some potential means of doing so are unsafe and/or dangerous. Third, they can enhance performance courageously by withstanding those institutional pressures and external rewards that contradict the internal goods of sport or lower them in priority below the external goods bestowed by the institutions.

It must be noted that the material Scott has presented in his paper is pregnant with possibilities for additional research. And, as suggested in the latter part of my reaction, much productive research in answering the questions generated by his paper would involve ethicists in cooperation with sport physiologists, biomechanists, psychologists, and pedagogues. Such research efforts would be similar in principle to the kind of cooperative work now being done in medical ethics.

As indicated earlier in my remarks, I have a disagreement with something I assume Scott intended. Recognizing that my assumption about Scott's intent could be in error, the disagreement must be identified so that Scott may react to it. Here is my disagreement: Without eliminating the significance of an ethic of virtue, I do not see how it is, by itself, capable of generating ethically appropriate actions in the enhancement of sport performance.

If you will recall my earlier contrast of an ethic of virtue with an ethic of duty, you will find "being" versus "doing." A person can be honest, courageous, and just and still not do what is ethically right in a given situation. Interestingly, an intellectual idiot can have the three cited virtues and still not do what is ethically best in a given situation. This is because such virtues *dispose* a person to act in honest, courageous, and just ways but they do not tell him or her what is the ethically best action.

Accordingly, an adequate ethic requires an ethic of duty composed of rationally argued and stated principles, maxims, or guides for use in decisions. Nonetheless, a complete ethic would find an important function for both virtue and duty. Duty would provide the content for ethical actions while virtue would provide the driving motives and intentions for doing what must be done *willingly*. Thus, duty would not be disagreeable in the way Ogden Nash implied in his "Kind of an Ode to Duty"

> *Oh duty, why hast thou not*
> *the visage*
> *of a sweetie or a cutie?*

President's Address — 1991

Roberta J. Park
University of California, Berkeley

I hope you will permit me to deviate a little from the usual President's Address and extend to you a personal welcome from the city by the Golden Gate. This region is historically renowned for its multicultural populations as well as its scenic beauty. It also has a rich and diverse sporting heritage. When 49ers, lured by the promise of gold, arrived in northern California, the indigenous population was estimated to be 500 inhabitants. The numerous small tribes of Native Americans engaged in pastimes such as stick dice and hoop and pole. With the arrival of Spanish-speaking missionaries as well as settlers from Mexico, events such as *correr el gallo* and *colea el toro* (a local version of bullfighting) became popular.

The first sporting organization was the San Francisco Cricket Club, founded in 1852 by Her Majesty's British Consul. It was also in 1852 that the San Francisco Turnverein was established by a group of local German and German-Jewish residents, many of whom had fled the uprisings of 1848 in their native country. (Among the founding members was Charles Krug, a name now famous for its association with California wine.)

By the 1860s, there were scores of sports and recreations for local residents. Most were ethnically oriented, reflecting the city's multicultural population. The Germans, Irish, Swiss, and Italians all had militia companies that held regular marksmanship contests in which high performance standards prevailed. They also sponsored frequent picnics at which simple games were played. The Brannan Guards, a local Black militia company, featured a game of "baseball" at its 1873 gathering.

Although baseball had been known to locals in the 1850s, it was the 1869 visit of the Cincinnati Redstockings (the first avowedly professional baseball team) that catapulted the game into widespread favor. (A third match between an "all star" California cricket team and one from Vancouver, British Columbia, was never played, as men turned avidly to "the American Game.") By the 1880s and 1890s, as in other parts of the nation, newspapers in northern California were filled with box scores, accounts of local baseball games, and stories of the outstanding performances of the players.

Local residents also played soccer, a game that was especially popular among arrivals from the British Isles. Between the two world wars, extensive soccer leagues (with teams representing at least a dozen nationalities) regularly held matches at Golden Gate Park. The standard of performance at many of these matches was described as excellent.

When the University of California moved to its Berkeley location in 1873, the students began to play desultory soccer-like football games among themselves. Soon they began to arrange matches with local high schools and with the Olympic Club. The Olympic Club had been founded in 1860 (8 years before the New York Athletic Club) by a group of young men practicing gymnastics in the backyard of the Nahl brothers. They had become quite accomplished gymnasts and wanted to exercise and socialize in surroundings that were more congenial than Frank Wheeler's local gymnasium and boxing arena.

The Olympic Club fostered a great deal of high-level sporting competition in the late 1800s. Its president, William Greer-Harrison, played an important role in the local conversion from American football to rugby following the death of a player in the 1905 NYU–Union College game. When Stanford University opened in 1891, athletic contests were immediately arranged with the University of California. "The big game," as the annual football contest came to be known, was the gala athletic and social occasion of the fall season.

In response to increasing criticisms of football, the presidents of both universities became convinced that the game must be transformed or abandoned. Dissatisfied with the modest changes that were being discussed in the East, they pursuaded their institutions to adopt rugby. The game was never popular with players, or with alumni who had played the American version. Gridiron football returned during World War I, largely because it was believed to be of great value in improving the physical performance of the fighting man.

Competitions for women at the two local universities were also established during the 1890s. Walter Magee, Associate in Physical Training at the University of California, had traveled east to investigate the latest developments. He returned with the game of basketball and immediately taught it to the young women at Berkeley. The first extramural game was played in 1892 between a team from the University of California and one from Miss Head's School.

Four years later, young women from Berkeley crossed San Francisco Bay by ferryboat to meet a team from Stanford University at the San Francisco Armory. The young men who had accompanied the players were left at the door, as it would have been unseemly to engage in an athletic contest before a "mixed" crowd. The final socre was 2–1, which makes me think that both teams would have benefitted from having their performance enhanced.

This, perhaps, is a good place to draw this little digression to a close and turn briefly to current concerns and to issues that will be discussed during these 1991 meetings. As you know, the question of future directions, and a possible name change, for the American Academy of Physical Education has been a topic of considerable interest and debate in recent years. We will have an opportunity to examine this matter in considerable depth.

Meanwhile I would like to pick up on a highly significant point that George Sage (1991) made in the paper that closed the formal program of the 1990 Academy meetings. The title of that paper, you may recall, was "Paradigms, Paradoxes and Progress: Reflections and Prophecy." Having sketched the shifting emphases that have characterized American physical education over the last century, George cogently observed,

> But paradigmatic hegemony is never guaranteed. The structure of academic
> disciplines and professional programs of study and training are not static,

and trends are not random processes. There are structured moments for intellectual enterprises in which alliances shift, older constellations are displaced, and new views arise. One of those structured moments began in college and university departments of physical education in the 1960s and gained momentum in the 70s. . . . This movement was spearheaded by young scholars wishing to promote and advance the disciplinary study of human movement. (p. 156)

We might, I think, say that these young scholars—and not a few older ones for that matter—were enhancing human performance: performance in the many and varied interweaving threads of science and scholarship upon which our field must be built if it is to flourish and grow in the face of the academic demands of the 1990s. The famous anthropologist Victor Turner (1974), building upon a concept put forth early in this century by the Dutch anthologist Arnold Van Genep, has applied the concept of *liminal* and *liminoid* to human cultures. From the Latin for "threshold," *limen* signifies, for Turner, an important phase in which one is transformed from one state (or status) to another.

The implication is that one moves to a higher or more advanced status. I view the phase our profession has been in for the last several years as being tantamount to liminal—or better, liminoid—by which Turner means something slightly more complex than liminal. This stage is characterized by uncertainty, often confusion, from which one may emerge having seen new possibilities.

I think this is an important step, one from which we must now extract ourselves. From the "buzzing confusion" of being "in limbo," we must emerge with clearer visions. We must now sharpen our focus, delineate the essential elements, define the new possibilities, and move forward, taking from our past that which is best while abandoning, even though we may still respect, that which will no longer serve our collective purposes. If we do, our future can be bright indeed. If we do not, our future is problematic.

The mathematician turned philosopher turned educator, Alfred North Whitehead (1929), reflected on this condition many years ago in a slim book entitled *The Aims of Education*. From wherever a learner is, she or he gathers new information, typically to the extent that all becomes a buzzing confusion. Further exploration and reflection, however, enables the individual to emerge on the upward spiral (which is Whitehead's metaphor) of knowledge with the realization that he or she has returend, *not* to the same place but to deeper and broader understandings.

If we apply this to our current circumstances, we may find we have enhanced our performance in dealing with ideas—and ideas, in the long run, are what higher education is all about. In physical education, however, we have the added advantage of very often being able to put ideas into practice!

As we participate in the discussions that comprise the formal program, let each of us sympathetically and continually ask, What does this small slice of our large field contribute to *my* vision of it? What might I bring from my own research and practice, from my own unique perspective, that draws this into a larger and more meaningful whole? What exciting new ideas and opportunities does this elicit? Let us each ask ourselves, Where am I on the spiral of my own learning? How does this, then, fit into a larger whole of the evolution of our field—a field to which many, possibly most, of us here have given 20, 30, or more years of dedicated service? Let us ask singly, and collectively, how might each of us contribute to enhancing the performance of our field?

References

Sage, G.H. (1991). Paradigms, paradoxes, and progress: Reflections and prophecy. In R.J. Park & H.M. Eckert (Eds.), *The Academy Papers: New possibilities, new paradigms?* (No. 24, pp. 154-161). Champaign, IL: Human Kinetics.

Turner, V. (1974). Liminal to liminoid in play flow and ritual: An essay in comparative symbology. *Rice University Studies,* **60**(30), 53-92.

Whitehead, A.N. (1929). *The aims of education and other essays.* New York: Macmillan.

PRESIDENTS

American Academy of Physical Education

*1926-30 Clark W. Hetherington
*1930-38 Robert Tait McKenzie
*1938-39 Robert Tait McKenzie
         Mabel Lee
*1939-41 John Brown, Jr.
*1941-43 Mabel Lee
*1943-45 Arthur H. Steinhaus
*1945-47 Jay B. Nash
*1947-49 Charles H. McCloy
*1949-50 Frederick W. Cozens
*1950-51 Rosalind Cassidy
 1951-52 Seward C. Staley
*1952-53 David K. Brace
*1953-54 Neils P. Neilson
*1954-55 Elmer D. Mitchell
 1955-56 Anna S. Espenschade
*1956-57 Harry A. Scott
*1957-58 Charles C. Cowell
*1958-59 Delbert Oberteuffer
*1959-60 Helen Manley
 1960-61 Thomas E. McDonough, Sr.
*1961-62 M. Gladys Scott
 1962-63 Fred V. Hein
*1963-64 Carl L. Nordly
*1964-65 Eleanor Metheny
 1965-66 Leonard A. Larson
*1966-67 Arthur A. Esslinger
 1967-68 Margaret G. Fox
*1968-69 Laura J. Heulster

1969-70 H. Harrison Clarke
1970-71 Ruth M. Wilson
1971-72 Ben W. Miller
1972-73 Raymond A. Weiss
1973-74 Ann E. Jewett
1974-75 King J. McCristal
*1975-76 Leona Holbrook
1976-77 Marvin H. Eyler
*1977-78 Louis E. Alley
1978-79 Marguerite A. Clifton
1979-80 Harold M. Barrow
1980-81 Aileene S. Lockhart
1981-82 Earle F. Zeigler
1982-83 Edward J. Shea
1983-84 Henry J. Montoye
1984-85 David H. Clarke
1985-86 G. Alan Stull
1986-87 Margaret J. Safrit
1987-88 Robert J. Malina
1988-89 Waneen W. Spirduso
1989-90 Charles B. Corbin
1990-91 Roberta J. Park
1991-92 Robert W. Christina
        (current)
1991-92 Jerry R. Thomas (elect)

---

*Deceased

THE AMERICAN ACADEMY OF PHYSICAL EDUCATION

The American Academy of Physical Education is an honorary organization composed of individuals who have made significant contributions to the field of physical education.

When the American Academy of Physical Education was officially founded in 1930 there were 29 charter fellows, including four women (Jessie Bancroft, Amy Morris Homans, J. Anna Norris, M.D., Elizabeth Burchenal), and 12 medical doctors. R. Tait McKenzie was elected the first president and served as such until his death in 1938. When the constitution was adopted on December 31, 1930, the total number of *Active Fellows* (who constituted the governing body of the Academy) was set at 50. Since then the total number of Active Fellows has been raised to 125. Additionally, *Corresponding Fellows* are professionals in other countries who have rendered outstanding service to physical education; *Associate Fellows* are individuals in related fields who have rendered outstanding service to the field. *Fellows in Memoriam* (Gulick was the first named) and *Fellows Emeriti* have been added.

In 1930 the Academy began to hold annual meetings. Since 1951 the Academy has published its annual proceedings and papers, *The Academy Papers* (first published in 1963). The majority of annual Academy meetings are open upon payment of a nominal registration fee. As a professional contribution to Alliance members, the Academy sponsors the R. Tait McKenzie Memorial Lecture at the annual meeting.

Over the years the Academy has honored individuals with a variety of awards. Amy Morris Homans received the first Honor Award in 1931. The Hetherington Award, the highest honor that the Academy makes to one of its retired members, has been awarded regularly since 1956. Organizations and agencies that have conducted outstanding programs or projects significant to physical education receive citations.

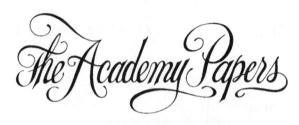

With comprehensive coverage of current topics and contributions from the foremost scholars in the field, *The Academy Papers* are invaluable resources for every physical education professional and student.

New Possibilities, New Paradigms?, Volume 24
Roberta J. Park, PhD, and Helen M. Eckert, PhD, Editors
Nineteen papers take an introspective look at the present and future of research issues and pedagogical concerns in physical education and the sport sciences.
1991 • Paper • 176 pp • Item BPAR0313 • ISBN 0-87322-313-6

The Evolving Undergraduate Major, Volume 23
Charles B. Corbin, PhD, and Helen M. Eckert, PhD, Editors
Fifteen papers explore the evolving body of knowledge in physical education, the physical education profession, the name of the undergraduate major, teacher certification, and careers in exercise, movement, and sport.
1990 • Paper • 112 pp • Item BCOR0278 • ISBN 0-87322-278-4

Physical Activity and Aging, Volume 22
Waneen W. Spirduso, PhD, and Helen M. Eckert, PhD, Editors
1989 • Paper • 208 pp • Item BSPI0220 • ISBN 0-87322-220-2

Physical Activity in Early and Modern Populations, Volume 21
Robert M. Malina, PhD and Helen M. Eckert, PhD, Editors
1988 • Paper • 120 pp • Item BMAL0180 • ISBN 0-87322-180-X

The Cutting Edge in Physical Education and Exercise Science Research, Volume 20
Margaret J. Safrit, PhD, and Helen M. Eckert, PhD, Editors
1987 • Paper • 136 pp • Item BSAF0098 • ISBN 0-87322-098-6

Effects of Physical Activity on Children, Volume 19
G. Alan Stull, EdD, and Helen M. Eckert, PhD, Editors
1986 • Paper • 174 pp • Item BSTU0049 • ISBN 0-87322-049-8

Limits of Human Performance, Volume 18
David H. Clarke, PhD, and Helen M. Eckert, PhD, Editors
1985 • Paper • 144 pp • Item BCLA0099 • ISBN 0-931250-99-4

Exercise and Health, Volume 17
Helen M. Eckert, PhD, and Henry J. Montoye, PhD, Editors
1984 • Paper • 160 pp • Item BECK0056 • ISBN 0-931250-56-0

10   37

Human Kinetics Books
A Division of Human Kinetics Publishers, Inc.